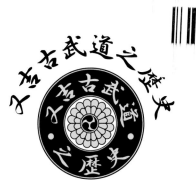

又吉古武道之歷史

## Andrea Guarelli

又吉古武道之歷史

# Okinawan Kobudō
## The History, Tools, and Techniques
## of the Ancient Martial Art

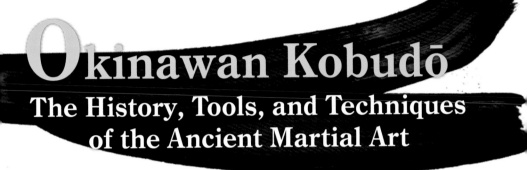

# Okinawan Kobudō

## The History, Tools, and Techniques of the Ancient Martial Art

**Master Andrea Guarelli**

**Translated by Sara Sturman**

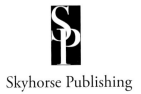

Skyhorse Publishing

Visit our website at www.skyhorsepublishing.com.

10 9 8 7 6 5 4 3 2

Library of Congress Cataloging-in-Publication Data is available on file.

Cover design by Radana Bandovà
Cover photo credit: Sensei Andrea Guarelli

Print ISBN: 978-1-63450-484-3
Ebook ISBN: 978-1-63450-962-6

Printed in China

# Disclaimer

The techniques illustrated in this volume are dangerous and they should be practiced exclusively under the supervision of a qualified Okinawan Kobudō teacher.

The author declines any responsibility for injuries incurred by readers who practice without qualified supervision.

To my teacher Matayoshi Shinpō:

A Master is like a swimming pool where you can learn to swim.

When you reach it, whole ocean is yours.

*Asan di Basra, Sufi Master*

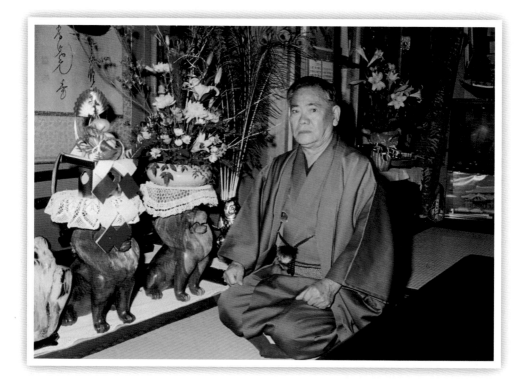

# Table of Contents

# Preface by Shinsei (Yasushi) Matayoshi

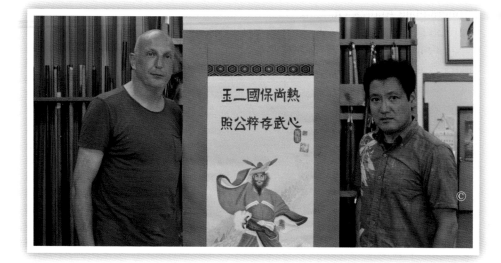

序文

この度は、父眞豊の直弟子である、アンドレア グアレッリ先生が、当流の歴史、技法、型、特に津堅赤人のウェーク手の教本をイタリア国にて出版されるとの事おめでとうございます。

父が亡くなりもう十七年になりますが、毎年のように、グアレッリ先生は、沖縄の我が家の仏前へお参りしてくださいます。 国や言葉の違いは、同じ武道を志す者には隔たり無く、父、祖父、家族への愛と尊敬に感謝の気持ちで一杯です。又、空手古武道の修行に中国へも度々行かれ、その類まれな探求心に、尊敬の念をいだいております。

數多くの空手の先生方のおかげで世界中に又吉古武道を修行者は、増えております。そのいっぽうでスポーツ化や組織の多様化等で父の心配していた本物の技や本部の必要性は、より難しくなります。 それでも貴重な直弟子である者達は誇りと自覚、責任を持って 光道館 道場訓

武を磨かんと欲さば

先ず心を磨け

心正しからざれば

武もまた正しからず

心を磨く道なり

父の言葉を心に刻み 生涯、武道、生き方を通して後世の者に數多くの歴史や技、真理の向上に、尽力してくださり、イタリア古武道協会及び又吉古武道の発展を心より願っております。

又吉眞靖(靖)

金硬流17代宗家

光道館道場館長

大日本武德會沖縄県支部長

財団法人日本古武道協會正会員

沖縄県空手道連合会 理事

I congratulate Andrea Guarelli Sensei, direct student of my father Shinpō, on the publication of his book about the history, techniques, and kata of our school, most of all the kata Chikin Akachu no ēku-di. Despite the seventeen years that have passed since my father's death, Guarelli Sensei comes every year to visit the Buddhist altar situated in our house in Okinawa. In spite of national and language differences, no distance exists between people who aspire to the same martial way (budō) and I am deeply grateful for his love and respect towards my father, grandfather, and family. Furthermore, I respect him for his extraordinary spirit of research, in fact he travels often to China to train his Karate and Kobudō.

Thanks to many Sensei, Matayoshi Kobudō practitioners are growing all over the world. At the same time, sport "drift" and differences between associations make the need to preserve original techniques and the dojo headquarters more difficult—something my father cared about very much. In spite of these difficulties, I direct students to refer to the Kōdōkan's Dōjō-kun:

"If you desire your combat art will be bright,
First purify your heart, if your heart is right,
also your combat art will be.
The Way is to purify your heart."

and to take my father words to heart.

I hope they will transmit to future generations the history and techniques with proud, consciousness and responsibility, through Budō and lifestyle, and by pursuing improvement of the truth.

I sincerely wish all the best in the development of A.I.K.O and Matayoshi Kobudō school.

*Shinsei (Yasushi) Matayoshi*
*Kingai-ryū XVII Sōke (leader)*
*Kōdōkan Dōjō director*
*Dai Nippon Butokukai director, Okinawan section*
*Japanese National Association of martial arts member*
*Okinawan Karatedō confederation councilor*

## PREFACE BY THE AUTHOR

My teacher, Shinpō Matayoshi, dedicated his entire life to the study and diffusion of Kobudō of Okinawa.

He studied with his father Shinkō and he traveled in China collecting a vast technical knowledge he passed along to his students.

He was a great businessman in real estate, and he dedicated much of his time to his great passion. In this way, it was very difficult to transmit wholly to his students all of what he knew. So he decided, very wisely, to split his knowledge among different students, so he could transmit the most amount of specific information possible without overloading each student. Then, students would share with the others what they had learned.

I have met all of the most important students of master Matayoshi and I noticed that, unfortunately, many years after his death, this full sharing of knowledge hasn't yet taken place. Strict rules have kept this from happening. For example: if a younger training student (kōhai) knew a kata that an older student (senpai) didn't know, the senpai would have been unlikely ask the younger student to teach it to him.

The strict relationship between kōhai/senpai seemed to prevent a back and forth flow of information. For this reason, nowadays, many of the most advanced students of the master don't know the school program entirely.

Personally, because of my thirst for knowledge and my desire to learn wholly the Matayoshi system, I never let barriers like that stop me. If somebody knew something I didn't, I absolutely had to ask him to teach me! However, Shinpō Matayoshi didn't teach all he knew.

The program illustrated in this book: Ryūkyū buki-jutsu, Kingai ryū, and Go Kenki denrai is very wide and only a part has been transmitted to practitioners.

My teacher widely taught the Ryūkyū buki-jutsu part, while the remaining techniques have been transmitted differently through the different students. Also the Kingai ryū program has been partly transmitted: kata Ueshi and Gojunana have been taught only to a few uchi-deshi of Kōdōkan Dōjō.

Nunti, tinbē, and suruchin techniques have been integrated into the form which is taught currently, while the other techniques and kata have never been taught.

The Go Kenki program has been transmitted partly: kata Hakkaku has been taught only to some students of Kōdōkan Dōjō, in particular to Yoshiaki Gakiya and Kenichi Yamashiro. They have taught it to only few people.

Master Matayoshi used to show this kata in public but never in the original version. He didn't want the whole form to be filmed and superficially transmitted.

Shinpō Matayoshi learned Saru-ken 猿拳 (monkey style) and Suiken 醉拳 (drunken style) techniques during his travels in Taiwan; they have been shown in public but have never been taught to anyone else.

Today it is clear that what the master didn't transmit to his students is lost forever. Consequently, the program we have today for the practice and investigation is only what he has taught us directly.

Training directly with master Matayoshi, with his greatest students, and thanks to many trips to Okinawa for the purpose of improvement and comparison (twenty-two trips to date) and to Fujian (China), I have grasped a vast technical knowledge to share with my students, uchi-deshi, and soto-deshi. The purpose of the A.I.K.O. (Italian Association Kobudō of Okinawa) and honbu dōjō Junshinkan has been to transmit this integral teaching program for more than two decades through new teaching and training methods, most of all in pairs. Most importantly, these exercises strictly preserve the original kata transmitted by the Matayoshi family for future generations.

*Andrea Guarelli*
*Junshinkan Dōjō technical director*
*A.I.K.O. Italian Association Kobudō of Okinawa President*
*I.M.K.A. International Matayoshi Kobudo Association President*
*O.K.I. Okinawan Karatedō of Okinawa technical director*
*Yongchun Baihe quan (12a generation) Italian section President*

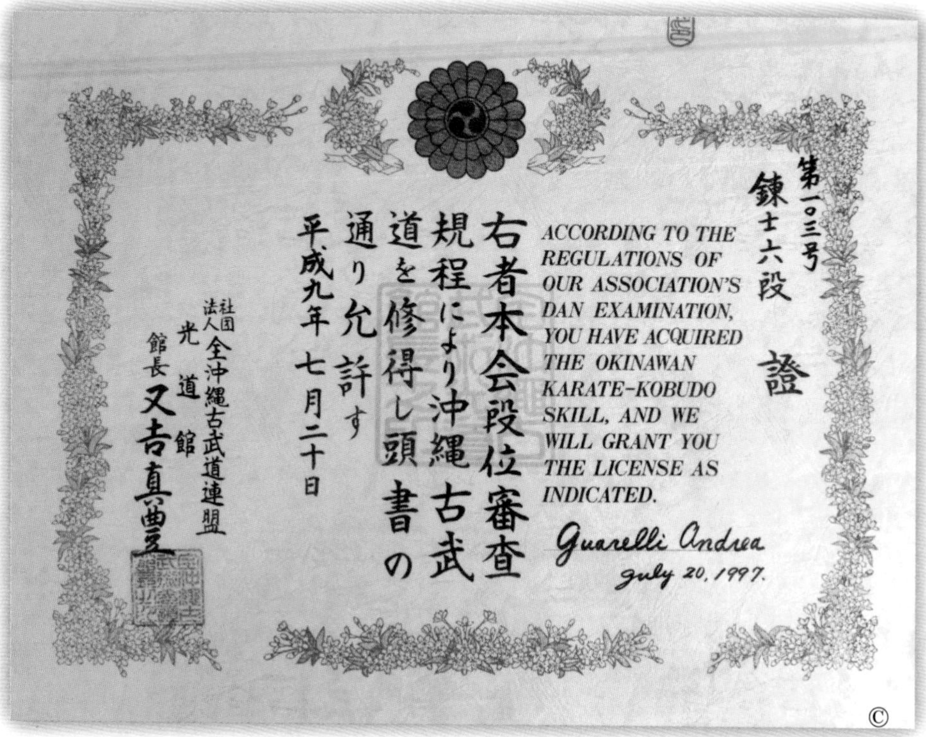

右者本会段位審査規程により沖縄古武道を修得し頭書の通り允許す

平成九年七月二十日

社団法人 全沖縄古武道連盟

光道館

館長 又吉真豊

第一〇三号

錬士六段

證

ACCORDING TO THE REGULATIONS OF OUR ASSOCIATION'S DAN EXAMINATION, YOU HAVE ACQUIRED THE OKINAWAN KARATE-KOBUDO SKILL, AND WE WILL GRANT YOU THE LICENSE AS INDICATED.

*Guarelli Andrea*
*July 20, 1997.*

**CERTIFICATE OF DEGREE AND QUALIFICATION**

Certificate n. 103 of 6° Dan - Renshi
Released to Andrea Guarelli
From Master Shinpō Matayoshi, on 20th July 1997.
The author, today is 8° DAN Kyōshi,
is the only European, and one of the few occidentals, who has received
this high degree and title directly by master Matayoshi.

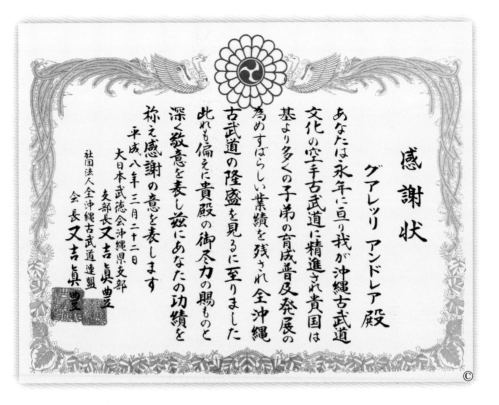

## CERTIFICATE OF THANKS

Mr. Guarelli Andrea, for a long time you have been applying yourself to the growth, diffusion and development, by your students in your country, of our cultural heritage which is Karate-Kobudō of Okinawa.
The extraordinary results you have reached have contributed to the prosperity of Zen Okinawan Kobudō Renmei.
To pay you tribute for your contribution in the association and to honor the result of your effort, I would like to demonstrate my gratitude.

*Matayoshi Shinpō*
*Dai Nippon Butokukai Okinawan-ken*
*Shibuchō (Okinawan delegation head of Dai Nippon Butokukai)*
*Shadan Hojin Zen Okinawan Kobudō Renmei Kaichō*
*(Zen Okinawan Kobudō Renmei President)*
*8° Year of Heisei era-3° month - 22° day*
*(22nd march 1996)*

# History of Matayoshi Kobudō

又吉古武道之歴史

# Introduction

The use of "white weapons" for self-defense has always been part of cultural heritage of the Ryūkyū Islands in Japan. In fact, one of the first terms used to define the martial arts of these islands was T*udi*, which didn't differentiate between techniques with weapons (*buki-jutsu*) and without weapons (*toshu-jutsu*). *Kobudō* and *Karatedō* according this point of view, were two wheels of the same axle, each one very important for the other. For people who practice *Karatedō* today, the study of weapons represents an opportunity to analyze historic free-hand techniques and their applications from a modern perspective.

The origin of the combat arts of Ryūkyū goes back to the period of the unification of the three kingdoms of Nanzan, Chūzan, and Hokuzan. The original combat systems of these islands and that of the Chinese which had been there for many years, fused with some Japanese techniques during the invasion of the archipelago by the Satsuma in 1609.

Akapeichin[1] Naoshiki (1721–1784) studied sword techniques of the *Jigen-ryū* school for many years, under the direction of Kuba Peichin Chito of *Ei* family and at the end he received a study certificate.

Eiso Naoyoshi also studied *Jigenryū*, such as *Naginata-jutsu* of the *Ten-ryū* school and he received certificates of these schools, which he took care of very jealously. However he prohibited his son to train in *yawara*[2] and "*karamutō*[3]

The original of what is here reported is taken from the article "Testament and last wills of Aka Naoshiki" from the *Okinawan Kokon* by Higaonna Kanjun (Higaonna Kanryu's son, famous *Tudi* expert). Also *Mastumura Sōkon,* a well-known *bushi* who lived in 1800, studied sword techniques of *Jigen-ryū* school.

During the first decades of the last century, an unknown Okinawan master introduced in Japan while neglecting, for practical reasons, the practice of *Kobudō*. The relationship between these two disciplines has now been forgotten, with the result that while *Karatedō* is very popular all over the world, *Kobudō* remains almost unknown. Fortunately, contrary to what had been happening in those years in Japan, in Okinawa some *Kobudō* experts had been teaching original techniques even to the present. Moreover, from the mid-twentieth century, *Okinawan Karatedō* began to be codified in "*ryu*," or school with a formal lineage, and also for *Kobudō*.

---

1    *Pēchin:* title in the Ryūkyū reign hierarchy. Often it was the class of *Pēchin* to transmit combat arts in the Ryūkyū.

2    *Yawara:* fighting techniques from Japan which are the basis of *jūjutsu.*

3    Karamutō: archaic term, probably the set of techniques will become known like "tudi" and then "karate."

又吉古武道之歷史

Some schools, which are still there on the island, such as *Ryuei-ryū Kobudō, Motobu-ryū, Honshin-ryū, Yamane-ryū*, and *Ufuchiku Kobudō* are practiced marginally and they risk extinction; however, they remain an important part of the martial heritage of Okinawa, regardless of their restricted dissemination.

Unlike the aforementioned *ryū*, the Matayoshi Kobudō school developed on the island, and it attracted local practitioners, but it also began to create interest among students from *Karatedō* schools (*ryūha* and *kaiha*) which had not been practicing techniques with weapons.

The same has happened to the *Ryūkyū Kobudō* school created by Shinken Taira, student of Moden Yabiku, who founded the association for preservation and development of *Ryūkyū Kobudō* (*Ryūkyū Kobudō Hozon Shinkokai*), which is now internationally known.

However, it is appropriate to remember that the origin of the *Matayoshi* family technique is even older and more widespread in the world.

Most information contained in this book comes from my direct experience of the system with Shinpō Matayoshi in Okinawa, with Yoshiaki Gakiya, and with other students of Sensei Matayoshi with whom I associated for decades, as well as his son Shinsei (Yasushi) Matayoshi.

This book is a report of conversations with all these people, such as the transcription of answers to some of my direct questions about of content and history of the system. Furthermore, I had the opportunity to train directly with the master, to frequent his house and visit his family, so I could ask him very confidential information about the school, often in the presence of his wife Haruko (who died in October 2012). After the master died, she was the source of the most important historical memory of the school. I eventually published information about the system published in Japanese in conjunction with various events organized by Matayoshi school in Okinawa; particularly for the commemoration of the third anniversary of the death of Shinpō Matayoshi sensei. The commemoration was held at the Okinawa Convention Centre, and featured a great international demonstration. I was honorably invited to perform individually the *sansetsukon kata*, while some of my students performed the *Sanchō-sai kata*.

# *Origins*

The Matayoshi family came from Taisō Shinbu (Ufugushiku Aji) and it continued during Ryūkyū reign into the munchū[1] of Chinese family "Má 麻" which took residence in Okinawa in the XXI century and got the power in the south of the island. Into this family were the learned, technicians and military men.

Then the clan divided into the Gima, Ishimine, Tawada, Matayoshi, Toguchi, Tana, Matsumura families, etc.

Ufugushiku Shinbu (大城眞武) lived in the Ryūkyū between XIV and the beginning of XV century. His Chinese name (kara-naa[2]) was Má Pǔwèi (麻 普蔚) and his daughter Samekawa was King Shō Shishō's mother, whose son, Shō Hashi was the founder of the first Shō dynasty. He was the founder of "Má" family and he has been the first to use the character "shin" (眞), now modernized as "真," transmitted to each descendant male of the family.

Six generations later Gima Shinjō (Chinese name Má Pínghéng - 麻平衡) linear descendant of Ryūkyū royal family restored the prestige of the family. Shinjō Gima (儀間真常), also

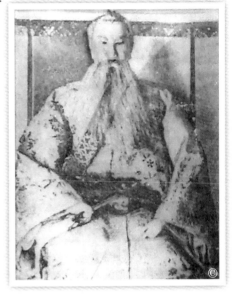

*Shinjo Gima's portrait*

called Mashi Shinjō Gima Oyakata[3], (1557-1644) gave an important contribution to the Island development. He was a noble of the Ryūkyū feudal government, an agricultural functionary and tutor of Sokan Noguni (野國總管), who brought the sweet potato from *Fujian* (China) in 1604. *Gima* took the vegetable his vassal brought with him and started to grow it. In a few years, sweet potato became one of the most important cultivation crops of the island. From Okinawa it was brought to Japan. *Gima* also imported and used sugar cane as a good of exchange. These two imported plants changed the course of Okinawa's history: the potato because it provided a high nutritional value and was suitable for the

---

1. *Munchū*: patriarch system of clan in *Ryūkyūs*.
2. Name system in use during *Ryūkyū* reign:
   a. *Warabi-naa*: infant name;
   b. *Yamatu-naa*: Japanese style name *(kamei*: surname - *ikai*: title/degree - *nanui*: name);
   c. *Kara-naa*: Chinese name (*sii*: surname - *imina*: name).

3. Title of the hierarchy of the *Ryūkyū* reign.

又吉古武道之歷史

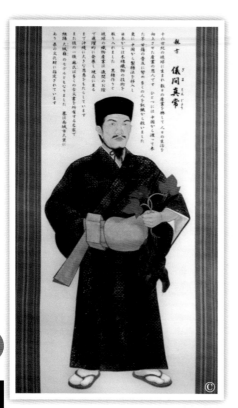

24 May 1786 in Okinawa and he was bestowed the title of *Sedo-zashiki*[3] in 1848, at the age of sixty-two.

By the time the Japanese *Meiji* government decided to integrate *Ryūkyūs* in the new prefectural system, some families of the city's *bujin* class lived in urban districts and farmers in the country. Moving was strictly prohibited, but there were some exceptions. An unemployed *bujin* was allowed to work as a farmer. For this reason, some of them moved to an agricultural area. These villages of *buijin*-farmers have been called *Yadoi*. It is here that we find the name of *Matayoshi Shintoku*: he has started to safeguard the combat arts of the *Matayoshi* family.

The fourteenth head of the family, *Matayoshi Shinchin*, (Chinese name *Má Shànshèn* - 麻善慎) father of *Matayoshi Shinkō*, was born on 15th November 1844 in Okinawa. In 1877 he was promoted to the rank of *Chikudun nu zashiki*[3].

He was teacher of tūdi and weapons and he collaborated with various contemporary experts.

He is one of the people, who contributed to the safeguard of the combat arts of *Ryūkyūs*.

climate and sugar cane because it represented a valuable good of exchange; both helped development of the island economy. Gima and Noguni were very popular on the island, both in life and after their death, so much that in 1937 a monument was built in their honor in the Naha park, to remember their contribution to Okinawa. In 1959 Gima's grave was removed by Cho Sumiyoshi to build an extension of an American military base, but it was rebuilt in 1993, thanks to state funds.

The thirteenth head of the family, Matayoshi Shintoku (Chinese name Má Kāiyuán - 麻開元) was born on

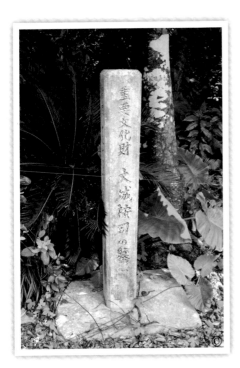

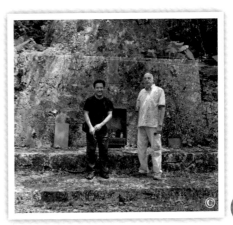

The author with Sōke Matayoshi Shinsei by the Ufugushiku Shinbu's grave.

23

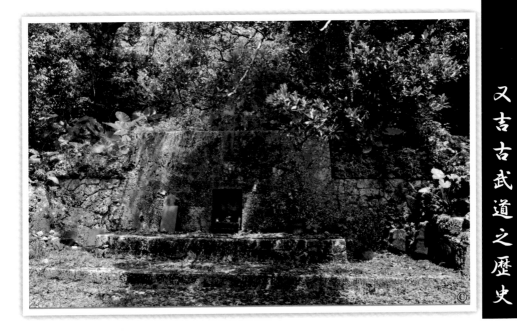

又吉古武道之歴史

# FAMOUS RELATIVES OF MÁ FAMILY

• Teruya Chikudun Pēchin Kanga (1786-1867), well known as Tūdi Sakugawa, was born in the Tunjumui district (now Torihori) a Shuri. He studied Chinese culture, language, and combat arts in China during the Qīng era. When he came back to Ryūkyūs he became professor at the Royal Academy. As a reward for his long and excellent service he was given an island in the Nakagusuku district where he became governor using the name of Sakugawa: for this reason his name was Tūdi Sakugawa. He is considered one of the founders of *Shurite*.

• Soeishi Ryōtoku (1772-1825) was an Oyakata and he created his own style, *bōjutsu*, which was acknowledged by the king of Ryūkyūs. He called "*Shiishi-nukun*" a kata of *bō* created by himself (*Soeishi-no-kon* in Japanese). After the abolition of the feudal clan system in favor of the prefectural system, the 8th patriarch of Soeishi family, Oyakata Ryōjutsu, taught his new techniques of *bō* and *Shiishi no kun kata* to Matayoshi Shinchin.

• Ishimine Chikudun Pēchin Shinchi was born on 1st May 1812 in Tunjumui village in Shuri and he died on 22nd December 1892. His Chinese name was Má Xíngrén (麻行仁), but he was better known as Tunjumui no bushi Ishimine "Ishimine the bushi of Tunjumui". Ishimine Shinchi was student of the famous Matsumura Sokon

and he left us a new version of *Passai kata*, in practice even today: *Ishimine no Passai*.

• Tawada Chikudun Pēchin Shinboku was born in 1814 in the Tunjumui village in Shuri and he died on 22nd December 1848 in Shuri, he was known also as Tawada no saki no Mēgantū and Tunjumui no saki no Tawada. Expert of *saijutsu*, at the age of nineteen he was chosen to give a demonstration of his talent in front of king Shō Kō. Tawada Shinboku created a *sai kata* still taught: *Tawada no sai*.

• Kuniyoshi Shinkichi was born in 1848 in the district of Kumoji in Naha (near Kume). He was also known as "Bushi Kunishi" in which "Kunishi" is the Okinawan pronunciation of "Kuniyoshi". Kuniyoshi learned Nahate with Sakiyama Chikudun nu Peichin Kitoku (1830-1914), who studied in China. When he was sixty years old, he moved to Nago, where he died in 1926.

又吉古武道之歴史

# 8 Shinko Matayoshi *(1888-1947)*

Matayoshi Shinkō was born in the Kakinohana district in Naha on 18th May 1888. He was the third son of Shinchin, he grew up in Shinbaru, near the Chatan village. As he was the only child to show a deep interest in martial arts, his father taught to him combat techniques of the family, with and without weapons; he also studied *bōjutsu* and *ēku-jutsu* (oar) with his grandfather Shintoku as well as learning *Chikin Akachu no ēkudi*, *Kubo no kon*, *Yonegawa no kon*, e *Yara no kon*. Then his father introduced him to Chokuhō Agena, a friend and a training partner from the village of Gushikawa, known also as Tiraguwa Gushikawa or Higa no tanmei.

*Agena* was an *Uēkata* of *Nishijō* in the village of Gushikawa where he was one of the guards. From Agena, Shinkō learned *sai* (trident) and *kama* techniques (reaping hook) and he widened his knowledge of *ēku* and *bō*. In *Yomitan* village he studied *nunchaku*, *tunkuwa*, *kurumanbō* (asymmetrical scourge) and *kuwa* (hoe) from a *bushi* called Irei Okina Shin'ushi (old Ire, known also as Moshigua Jitoudi) who lived in the village of Nozato for whom he was the head of the guards from 1885 to 1891.

During childhood, adolescence, and into his adulthood Shinkō Matayoshi concentrated only on martial arts. He continued to seek new masters and for this reason he struck up a friendship with

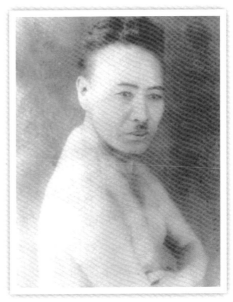

*Shinkō Matayoshi Sensei*

a Chinese merchant, Wu Xian Gui, called Go Kenki in the Japanese way.

Go Kenki was informed about a Chinese style of *kenpo*, *Baihe quan* (White Crane technique), and he shared his knowledge with Matayoshi. Shinkō had heard from his relatives and Go Kenki about the great Chinese martial arts, and with Go Kenki's encouragement he decided to go abroad to study them.

In the spring of 1905, at the age of seventeen, he left Okinawa for Hokkaido, and he planned to enter China through Manchuria. En route to Manchuria, which was an area rife with thieves, he passed through Hokkaido and Sakhalin and he joined a group of nomads for awhile. It is said that these nomads, who were also bandits, taught Shinkō to ride a

又吉古武道之歷史

---

*History and Techniques*

*Okinawan Kobudō*

horse, use a lasso, a sort of *suruchin* and other throw weapons (*shuriken*), because these techniques were fundamental for the group to hunt and fight. It was a very severe period in Shinkō's life, it was very hard and it is told that he learned a great deal about the combat art of the epoch.

After two or three years with that group (it is not clear how long he stayed in Manchuria), *Shinkō* moved south.

He stopped first in Shanghai, where he practiced a form of Chinese *Kenpo* for a certain period, although it's not clear what type it was. From there he moved back to his initial destination: the city of Fuzhou, in the Fujian region, arriving at Go Kenki's house. It was there he met Wu Jiao Gui (Go Koki) andWu Hian Gui (Go Kenki)'s father, from whom he started to learn *Kenpo* (probably *He quan*). Noticing young Shinkō's great abilities and passion for *Kenpo*, Wu Jiao Gui introduced him to a friend, a master known as Jin Ying (Kingai). Kingai was an old studious man and a martial arts master, and it is said he was a *senpai* of the same *Zhou Zhi He* (*Shushiwa* in Japanese, 1874-1926), who taught to Kanbun Uechi.

Kingai called his style *Kingai Nun*, or *Kingai-ryū* in Japanese (金硬流). He explained its name was a combination of two words meaning *Kin* (金) — "gold," or metal in a broad sense, and *Gai* (硬) – "strong," solid, like metal. Furthermore, the *Kin* character is the same as the master's name. The *Kingai-ryu* is often com-

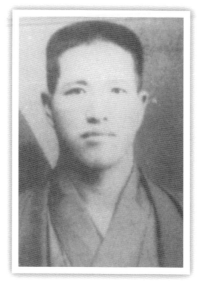

*Wu Xian Gui - Go Kenki Sensei (1887-1940)*

pared, ideologically, with the *Goju-ryu* principles for the purpose of contrast: the dualism of strong versus soft such as that of *Gōjū* of Okinawa. Kingai's teaching was very strict, but Shinkō dedicated himself briskly to the practice. Together with his martial studies, from Kingai he also learned acupuncture, medicinal Chinese moxa practices and herbal medicine. An important Kingai teaching, called *Cho Nin Ho*, was a method for hitting a man. This technique relied on precise knowledge of human anatomy and physiology to exactly hit a rival's vital points.

Shinkō came back to Okinawa between 1910 and 1918. In 1915 he was invited to demonstrate *Kobudō* in Tōkyō, it probably was the first demonstration of *Okinawan Kobudō* on the Japanese mainland. Then, around 1920, he established

又吉古武道之歴史

himself once again in Okinawa for many years.

By that time, he was practicing traditional Chinese medicine for the Okinawan community and during the same period he trained with Yamani Chinen (山根知念 1842-1925), Ryōkō Shiishi (添石良行 1852-1925), and Chojo Oshiro (大城朝恕 1887-1935), learning from them some new *Bō* techniques. In 1921, together with Chōjun Miyagi, he participated in a demonstration of martial arts in Ryūkyūs in honor of Prince Hirohito in the Shuri castle. In 1928 Shinkō participated in a demonstration in memory of Emperor Meiji in Tōkyō as an Okinawan prefectural representative; he showed *kama* and *tonfa* techniques while other master exhibited in *Karatedō*.He was awarded a medal by the government for his demonstration. Shinkō got married during the period he spent in Okinawa; his daughter Kimiko was born in 1919 and his son Shinpō in 1921. Around 1930 he came back to Fuzhou to meet again with his teacher Kingai in order to widen his studies, mostly focusing on weapons techniques: *tinbē*, *nunti*, *sansetsukon*, e *suruchin*. Before he came back again to Okinawa, master Kingai gave him a parchment, which is held today by the Matayoshi family; this is the parchment of Kōmyō Dai Gensui (Guāngmíng Dà Yuánshuài 光明大元师), protector God of Kingairyū. It is published and shown for the first time in this book. Shinkō came back to Naha in spring of 1934 and continued to work as a doctor of traditional Chinese medicine. He also started to teach the arts he had learned, developing them into the system that would become the Matayoshi Kobudō, as well as managing three dōjōs in Naha, Chatan, and Kadena. In addition to his son, his students included: Miyagi N., Hamamoto (theatrical actor), Shinjō H., Nakandakare, Omiya T., Kakazu M., Higa S., Kawakami S., Motobu S., Miyazato S., Iraha C.

He was deeply respected in the Okinawan martial arts community and he earned nicknames, such as Shinbaru Mateshi (Matayoshi of Shinbaru) and Kama nu ti Mateshi (Matayoshi of Kama). He died in May 1947, at the age of fifty-nine, and his death is considered a huge lost for the Okinawan martial arts community.

又吉古武道之歷史

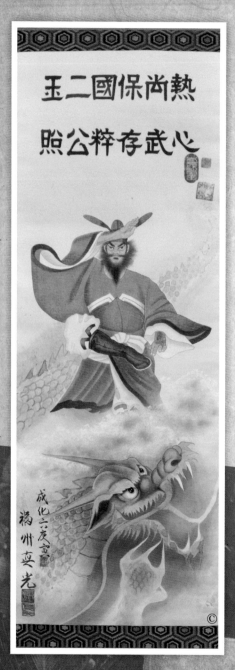

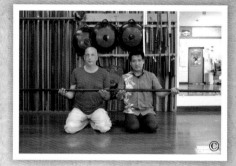

*The author and the present Sōke with the hasshaku-bō received from Shinjō Gima.*

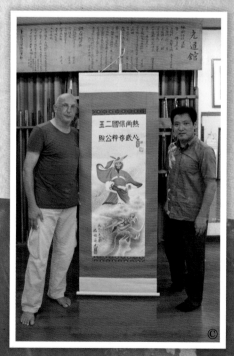

*The parchment Shinkō Matayoshi brought from China.*

# Shinpō Matayoshi

After Shinkō Matayoshi's death, the governance of the system he founded went to his son, Shinpō Matayoshi. Shinpō was born on 27th December 1921 in Kina, Yomitan. He started to train with his father when he was four years old. His father devoted himself to giving his son a martial arts education. In fact, he introduced his son to his friends and Budō colleagues. So Shinpō began to study with Chotoku Kyan (his mother's neighbor) in 1928, at the age of seven and for a short period, with his father's friend, Chōjun Miyagi and then with Seiko Higa, with whom he struck up a strong relationship.

(Master *Matayoshi* said to me once that "*Seiko Higa* was, for me, like second father.")

In 1935, he began training with his father's old friend, Go Kenki. Shinpō trained with him the end of the Second World War. In 1957 he moved to Kawasaki, in the Kanagawa prefecture, with many other Okinawans.

Life in Okinawa was very difficult after the war, and he moved to a highly industrialized region to earn his living. While he was in Kawasaki, he taught *Kobudō* to the Okinawan community and he practiced martial arts with some of the Okinawans who lived there. He returned to Okinawa in 1960, at which time he moved to a

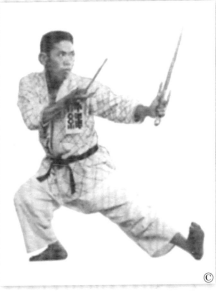

Photo of a young Shinpō Matayoshi Sensei.

small house behind Seiko Higa's *dōjō*. At first, he worked as a *sanshin* craftsman, a traditional string instrument of Okinawa. He was one of the most advanced students of Higa sensei and he taught *Kobudō* in Higa's *dōjō*, along with Shinken Taira and Kenko Nakaima. On December 27th 1962, Higa founded the Karate and Kobudō International Federation, and Shinpō became a member together with Shinken Taira, who became the vice president.

Shinpō remained at Higa's dōjō for years, teaching Kobudō in the dōjō, as well as outdoors and in many other places on the island. During his various moves through Okinawa, he knew many Kobudō practitioners, with whom he consulted about different aspects of the discipline.

又吉古武道之歴史

On these occasions he contacted some old students of his father, such as Mitsuo Kakazu. He traveled frequently to Taiwan, collecting a great number of traditional Chinese weapons. However, Shinpō lamented that the study of traditional weapons wasn't as popular as Karatedō, which was being taught widely.

He considered this a loss of the cultural and martial heritage of Okinawa, so he began to gather together many *Karatedō* practitioners to introduce them to the practice of *Kobudō*; then these people would have to share the teaching with their students.

On 17th October 1970 he founded the *Ryūkyū Kobudō Renmei Ryūkyūs Kobudō* Federation), a group dedicated to the practice and preservation of Okinawan weapons arts. In the same month, for the first Karate World Championship, which took place in Tōkyō's *Budōkan*, he showed the *ēku kata*. In 1972 (the year the United States returned Okinawa to Japan)

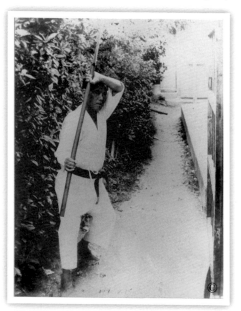

*The '60s — Exterior of Seiko Higa's dōjō (Shodōkan) with his ēku.*

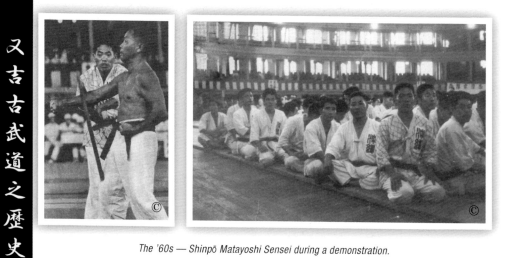

*The '60s — Shinpō Matayoshi Sensei during a demonstration.*

又吉古武道之歷史

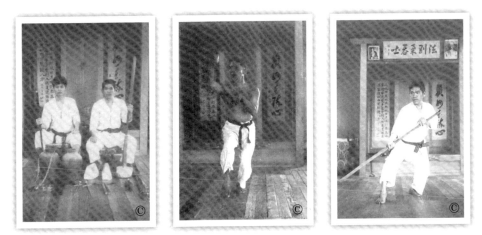

*The '60s — In Seiko Higa's dōjō (Shōdōkan) with Tetsuhiro Hokama (on the right) and executing Hakkaku (in the middle), with his ēku (on the left).*

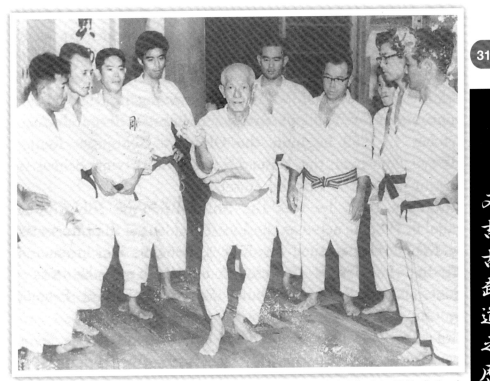

*The '60s — Master Seiko Higa while he was teaching kata Sēpai, on his right is Seiko Fukuchi (the first) and Shinpō Matayoshi (the third). On his left is Seikichi Higa's son (the second).*

又吉古武道之歷史

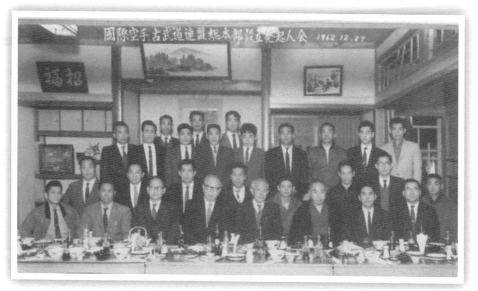

*December 27, 1962: foundation of the federation of which master Seiko Higa was president (Kokusai Karate Kobudō Renmei). On the first line, sat from left: Shinken Taira (the second), Seiko Higa (the fifth). On the second line sat from left: Chobuku Takamine (the second), Seiko Fukuchi (the third), Sekichi Odo and Sekichi Higa (the sixth and the seventh). On the third line standing from left: Shinpō Matayoshi (the fourth).*

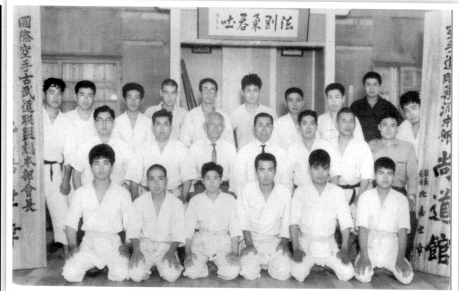

*1963 — Seiko Higa's dōjō, sat in the middle from left:
Seikichi Higa (Seiko's son), Seiko Fukuchi, Seiko Higa, Shinken Taira, Shinpō Matayoshi.*

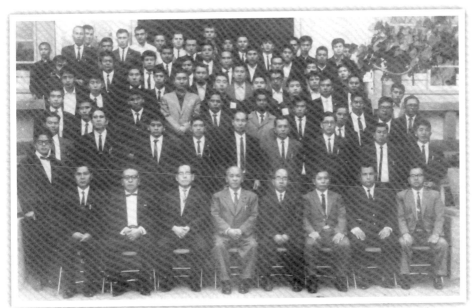

1967 — Meeting of the Zen Okinawan Karatedō Renmei. Sat on the first line from left:
Joen Nakazato (the first), Yuchoku Higa (the second), Shoshin Nagamine (the third), behind him is Shinpō Matayoshi,
Kanei Uechi (the sixth), Eiichi Miyazato (the seventh).

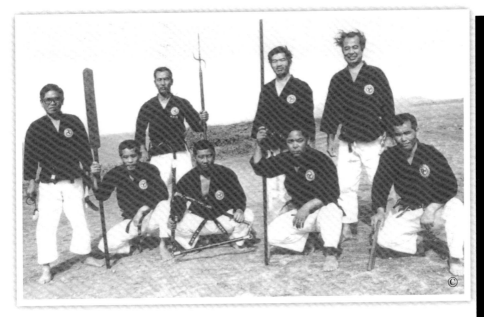

1968 — Master Matayoshi with some students for a service of the Japanese television:
Shoshin Miyahira, Shusei Maeshiro, Tsutomu Yamagawa, Takashi Kinjo, Koki Miyagi, and Seiko Itokazu.

又吉古武道之歴史

 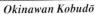

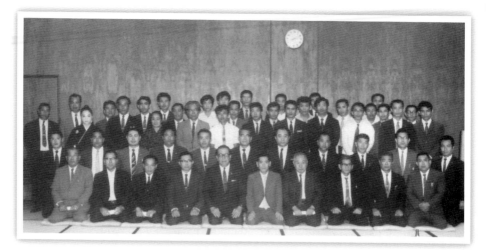

10/17/1970 — Foundation of the Ryūkyū Kobudō Renmei. There is: Shinpō Matayoshi (president), Chobuku Takamine, Kanei Uechi, Yuchoku Higa, Seiko Kina, Seiko Fukuchi, Seiko Itokazu, Kanei Katsuyoshi, Katsuya Miyahira, Koshin Iha, Sekichi Higa, Koki Miyagi, Tsutomu Yamagawa, Shusei Meshiro, Takashi Kinjo, and others.

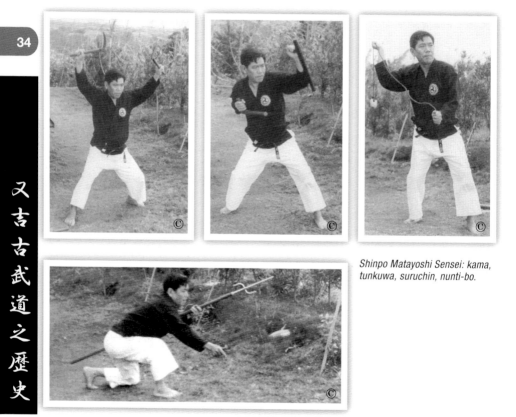

Shinpo Matayoshi Sensei: kama, tunkuwa, suruchin, nunti-bo.

又吉古武道之歷史

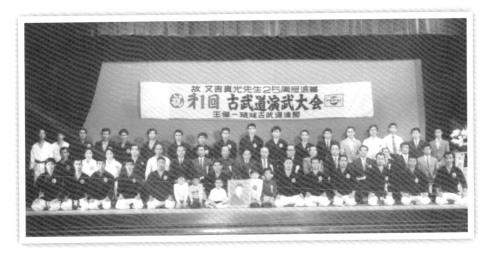

11/8/1971 — *The first demonstration of the Ryūkyū Kobudō Renmei Shinpō (25th anniversary of Shinkō Matayoshi's death). Seated in the middle Shinpō Matayoshi, in front of him, his son Shinsei.*

the organization changed its name to *Shadan Hojin Zen Okinawan Kobudō Renmei* or the Okinawan Kobudō Federation Co. Ltd (ZOKR) and received official acknowledgment in Okinawa and from the *Dai Nippon Butokukai*. In that same year, the first public demonstration by ZOKR was held, dedicated to the 25th anniversary of Shinkō Matayoshi's death. Some months later Shinpo Matayoshi went to Paris where, on the occasion of the second world championship of *Karate*, he demonstrated *Ēku* wearing a traditional Okinawan costume.

Shinpo became the first ZOKR President and he remained in charge for twenty-five years, until his death.

In the beginning, the ZOKR included his first dōjō students and some of Shinkō's students. Previous-

ly, Shinpō, with the help and advice of his earliest students, worked hard to codify both technical directives and exam programs for the future federation.

On March 1973, thanks to Roland Habersetzer's invitation, he taught a *Kobudō* seminar in Strasbourg, France. On that occasion, standing

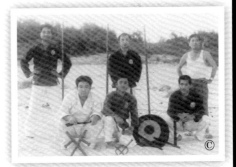

1982 — *Master Matayoshi on the Okinawan beach with some students. Between them there is Yoshiaki Gakiya (his successor), Kenichi Yamashiro and Koshin Kamura.*

又吉古武道之歷史

on a table so everyone could see, he demonstrated *nunchaku* techniques in front of 200 excited people.

Meanwhile his financial situation had improved and finally, in 1976, he could realize his dream: to have his own *dōjō* dedicated to the teaching of his school.

So, he bought a field in the district of Sobe in Naha and he built a new house for his family, in which in the ground floor was the *dōjō*, which he called *Kōdōkan* (光道館 or "place of the bright Way." The *kanji* "*kō*" (光), which means light or brightness, was taken from his father's name, Shinkō, to honor his memory.

Since his return to Okinawa in 1960, Shinkō Matayoshi had become an important person in the martial arts community of the island. He participated in public events about Okinawa and its *budō*, performing a demonstration during both the Kagoshima's gala and the Sport and Athletics Festival of Amami Oshima's island, both events to commemorate the reannexation of Okinawa to Japan.

His *dōjō* and the ZOKR kept a strict program of demonstrations, television appearances and other public displays during its history. He believed that Okinawan martial arts were part of the Okinawan culture

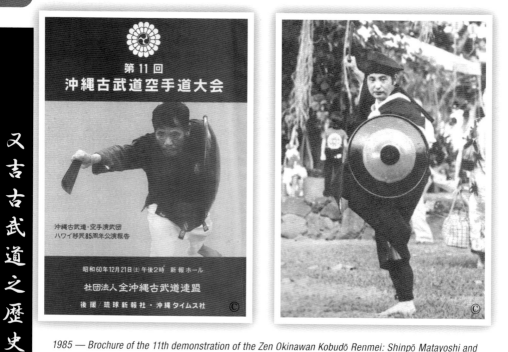

1985 — Brochure of the 11th demonstration of the Zen Okinawan Kobudō Renmei: Shinpō Matayoshi and Yoshiaki Gakiya with tinbē.

又吉古武道之歴史

and that they should keep their special relationship within the community, but also retain visibility. Up until his death he was very active in Okinawan organizations, in fact he was:

*Zen Okinawan Kobudō Renmei* (president, since its founding);

For Shinpō sensei, it was very important to maintain a connection between Japanese martial arts and their main organizations. He was the representative of the Dai Nippon Butokukai for the Okinawan prefecture, a position which was of Chōjun Miyagi, so the ZOKR and his dōjō were recognized by this organization. On 10th October 1987 he was officially recognized for his ability and his efforts to promote and preserve Okinawan martial arts, receiving the 10° Dan and the title of Hanshi from His Imperial Highness Higashi Fushimi Jigo, President of the Dai Nippon Butokukai. In that period he was also recognized as an important cultural treasure of the Butokukai, as well as member of the directive council. He was a member of the directive council of the *Nihon Kobudō Kyokai* Japan Traditional Martial Arts Association for many years. This organization, in Tōkyō's Budōkan, includes some of the most prestigious masters of traditional *Budō*.

At present, his son Shinsei (Yasushi) Matayoshi holds these positions.

As he shared his knowledge both in Okinawa and all over the world, Shin-

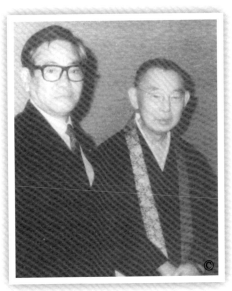

The master with His Imperial Highness reverend Higashi Fushimi Jigo, president of the Dai Nippon Butokukai.

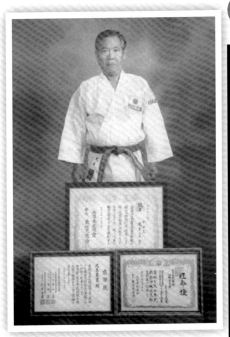

Shinpō Matayoshi with the acknowledgment of the Dai Nippon Butokukai.

又吉古武道之歴史

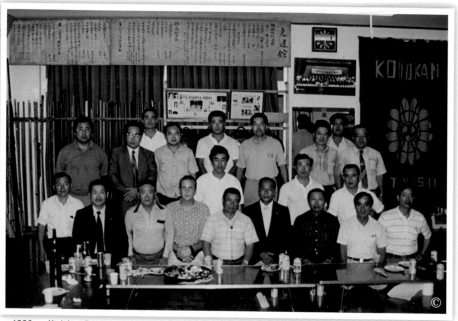

*1990 — Kōdōkan Dōjō, meeting of the Zen Okinawan Kobudō Renmei. Sat on the first line from left: Koshin Kamura, Shusei Maeshiro, Shinpo Matayoshi, Andrea Guarelli, Koki Miyagi, Shōshin Miyahira, Josei Yogi, Seiki Gibo, Isao Irei. The fourth standing on the left is Yoshiaki Gakiya.*

又吉古武道之歴史

pō sensei was crucial for the wide diffusion and the worldwide promotion of the *Okinawan Budō*. Like his fellow Okinawans, *Shinpō sensei*, loved his wonderful island and he believed deeply that there was a strict link between martial arts of Okinawa and the culture of his inhabitants, and that the international distribution of these arts would help to improve humanity by developing the psychophysical and moral aspects of those who practiced.

By founding the ZOKR he gave a great boost to the safeguard and promotion of Okinawan martial arts, teaching seminars and giving demonstrations in Japan and in many others countries.

Of note was the seminar he taught in Italy in 1995, in which he was assisted by the author of this book. Over the course of several days, Shinpō sensei taught the techniques of: *bō, sai, tunkuwa, nunchaku, kama, ēku*

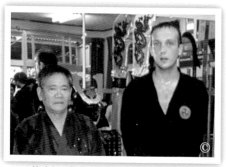

*Kōdōkan Dōjō: Shinpō Matayoshi Sensei and the author.*

*e sansetsukon*. Shinpō sensei and the author also trained together in the style of the White Crane, along with its applications.

He scrupulously handed down the traditional training methods, and he allowed his students to participate in competitions of *Kobudō* during the last years of his life.

He was considered a strict teacher, who shaped his students in *dōjō* training them intensely. However, he was open to changes in the world, welcoming new training methods that he and his students developed. He was also available both to share his art worldwide and to give hospitality in his *dōjō* to students coming from all over the world. Besides this, he was very passionate about local culture and he maintained contacts with the music and traditional dance communi-

ties. Some traditional dancers trained in *Kōdōkan*, and Shinpō helped them to introduce some *karatè* and *kobudō* techniques into their dances. Among his most important students were Mrs. *Hiroko Ogido*, a famous traditional dance teacher and expert of *Matayoshi Kobudō*. She collaborated with Eiko Miyazato to create *"himo kama no mai"* (reaping hook with string dance).

Sōke Matayoshi Shinpō died on September 7th 1997 in Naha, leaving his wife Haruko and his children Yasushi and Kiyomi.His death was a huge loss for the Okinawan martial arts community.

He will be remembered as one of the most important figures for the development of Okinawan martial arts after the Second World War and also for his great humanity. He left behind

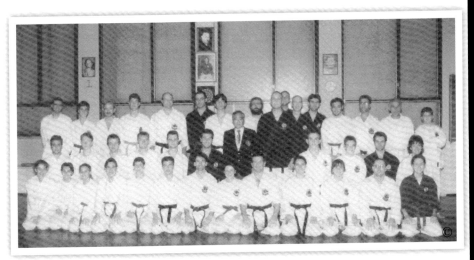

*Italy 1995 — Shinpō Matayoshi Sensei in the old Junshinkan Dōjō.*

又吉古武道之歷史

some expert students, who transmitted the teaching, while the formal and spiritual guide of the system (*sōke*) went to his son Shinsei.

Sōke Shinsei (Yasushi) Matayoshi was born in 1965, graduated from the International Business College, and is a real estate businessman. He doesn't personally practice *Okinawan Kobudō* but he is seriously involved in the management of Matayoshi's School and he has replaced his father in all his directive roles.

When master died, the rank of *Kanchō* of *Kōdōkan*, teaching and techniques responsible of the *dōjō*, went to Yoshiaki Gakiya, an inner disciple for more than twenty years. In the same period, the guide of ZOKR went to Shōshin Miyahira, who was a member for many years.

In 2001 Yoshiaki Gakiya left the *Kōdōkan*. Since then many assistants have succeeded him. In 2011 he had a cerebral hemorrhage with a consequent hemiparesis which prevented him from continuing to practice and teach *Kobudō*.

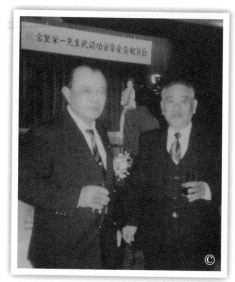

*My teachers together! Eiichi Miyazato and Shinpō Matayoshi.*

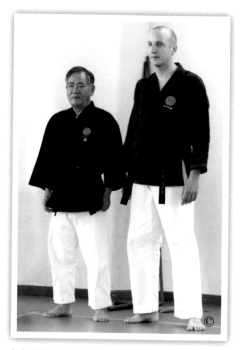

*Italy 1995— Shinpō Matayoshi Sensei with the author.*

〔新役員〕
沖縄古武術　金硬流　光道館総本部

会　　長　　又吉　春子　靖
顧問・相談役　宜保　成喜
顧　　問　　我喜屋　良章
理事長兼館長　早坂　義文
副理事長兼事務総長　香村　好信
常任理事兼事務局長　山城　健一
常　任　理　事　神谷　政光
理　　事　　伊敷　秀忠
書記・会計　大村　朝洋

※副理事長と常任理事は副館長を兼ねる。

September 1997 — Advice from Kōdōkan Honbu Dōjō about the new composition of the direction after Shinpō Matayoshi's death: Yasushi Matayoshi (son) president, Haruko Matayoshi (Shinpō's wife) and Seiki Gibo special councilors, Yoshiaki Gakiya president of the directive council and technical director, other councilor and secretaries Yoshifumi Hayasaka, Koshin Kamura, Kenichi Yamashiro, Masamitsu Kamiya, Hidetaka Ishiki, Tomohiro Omura.

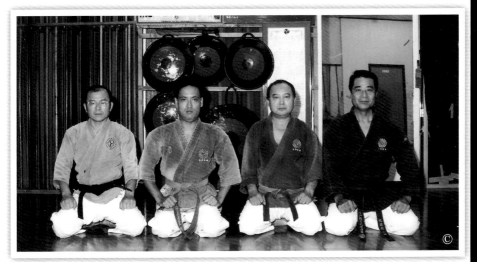

September 1997 — the direction of Kōdōkan after Shinpō Matayoshi's death: Koshin Kamura (teacher), Sōke Shinsei Matayoshi, Yoshiaki Gakiya (technical director), Kenichi Yamashiro (teacher).

又吉古武道之歴史

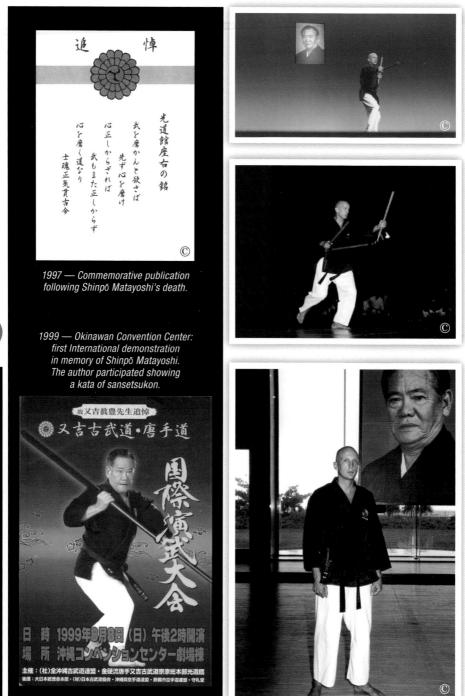

追悼

光道館座右の銘

武を磨かんと欲さば
先ず心を磨け
心正しからざれば
武もまた正しからず
心を磨く道なり
士魂正気貫古今

1997 — Commemorative publication
following Shinpō Matayoshi's death.

1999 — Okinawan Convention Center:
first International demonstration
in memory of Shinpō Matayoshi.
The author participated showing
a kata of sansetsukon.

故又吉眞豊先生追悼
又吉古武道・唐手道
國際演武大会
日　時　1999年8月8日（日）午後2時開演
場　所　沖縄コンベンションセンター劇場棟
主催：（社）全沖縄古武道連盟・金硬流唐手又吉古武道宗家総本部光道館
後援：大日本武徳会本部・（財）日本古武道協会・沖縄県空手道連盟・那覇市空手道連盟・守礼堂

又吉古武道之歴史

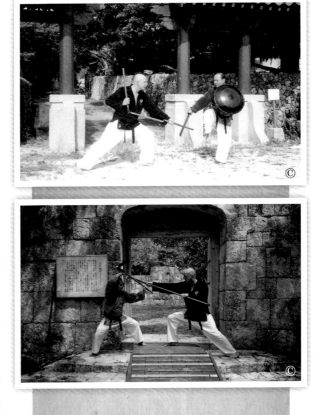

Below, two phone cards issued in his honor by NTT (Japanese telephone company).

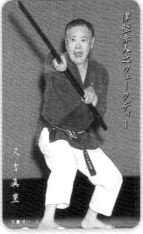

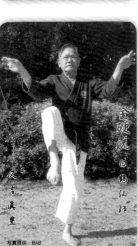

The author with Yoshiaki Gakiya in Okinawa:

*above, sansetsukon against tinbē and kuwa against nunti-bō*

*below, in Kōdōkan dōjō – some years earlier*

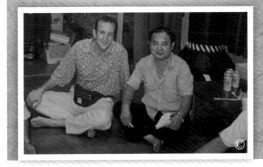

又吉古武道之歴史

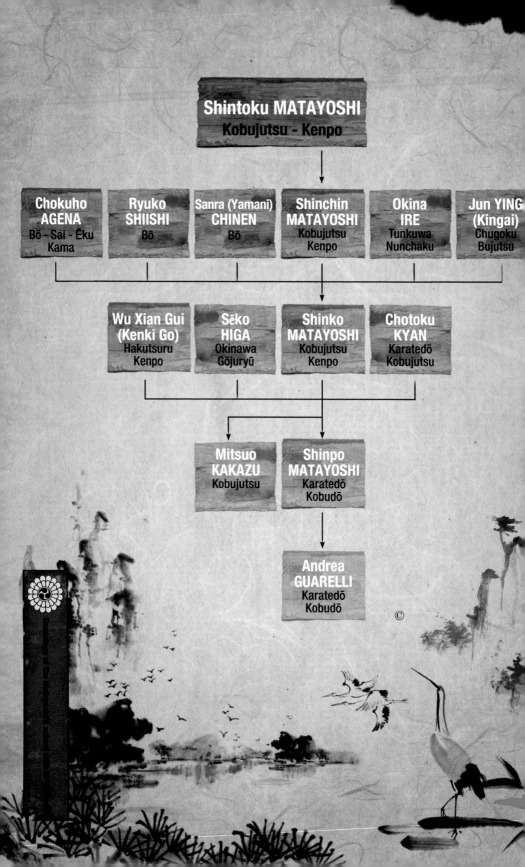

**Shintoku MATAYOSHI**
Kobujutsu - Kenpo

**Chokuho AGENA**
Bō - Sai - Ēku
Kama

**Ryuko SHIISHI**
Bō

**Sanra (Yamani) CHINEN**
Bō

**Shinchin MATAYOSHI**
Kobujutsu
Kenpo

**Okina IRE**
Tunkuwa
Nunchaku

**Jun YING (Kingai)**
Chugoku
Bujutsu

**Wu Xian Gui (Kenki Go)**
Hakutsuru
Kenpo

**Sēko HIGA**
Okinawa
Gōjuryū

**Shinko MATAYOSHI**
Kobujutsu
Kenpo

**Chotoku KYAN**
Karatedō
Kobujutsu

**Mitsuo KAKAZU**
Kobujutsu

**Shinpo MATAYOSHI**
Karatedō
Kobudō

**Andrea GUARELLI**
Karatedō
Kobudō

©

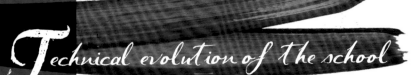

# Technical evolution of the school

The technical background of the *Matayoshi Kobudō*, as well as some other various ryu-ha, is composed by techniques taken from different origins.

The base technique of the system is founded on the martial arts of *Ryūkyū's* reign (*Ryūkyū Ōchō Jidai Kobujutsu*) that *Shinkō Matayoshi* studied following traditions of the family and includes *ēku-jutsu* of *Chikin Akachu* and classical forms of *Okinawan bō-jutsu*.

This also includes *sai*, *kama*, other techniques of *bō* and *ēku* of master *Agena*, *tunkuwa* and *nunchaku* of master *Irei* and then other forms of *bō* from *Yamani*, *Shiishi* and *Oshiro*. In addition to the original Okinawan elements, there are the techniques that Shinkō learned during his travels abroad in Manchuria, Shangai, and Fuzhou.

The White Crane of *Go Kenki* and various techniques with and without weapons were learned from master Kingai, including *nunti*, *tinbē*, *sansetsukon* and *suruchin*. These are the elements that Shinkō Matayoshi elaborated upon to create a uniform whole, which he transmitted to his students and to his son.

The development of the school has continued thanks to the work of Shinpō's son, who, like his father, many years before in Okinawa, had many different teachers.

From his father he learned various techniques of the Ryūkyū's reign period, as well as the teachings of Kingai.

Furthermore he studied *Karatedō* and *bō-jutsu* with Chotoku Kyan, Gōjūryu with Seiko Higa, and White Crane with Go Kenki, joining many technical exchanges with different Okinawan teachers, including his father's other students.

Shinpō, his students and his collaborators together formalized the *kata* system, they decided what had to be included and what was left out—they also created the base sequences for each of the weapons (*hōjōundo*).

For example, they selected only five *katas* of *bō* excluding others from the official list and from exam programs.

One difference from other schools is that in the practice of *Matayoshi Kobudō* training in pairs is a fundamental part; this is done with *kumiwaza* exercises and *kata bunkai* forms.

While the various *kata bunkai* of *bō* were made uniform, other weapons of the system have been developed by the various students of the master on their own, but under the master's supervision.

Moreover, some teachers have completed the program creating new base *katas* and exercises in pairs more suitable for the current teaching of the school.

45

又吉古武道之歴史

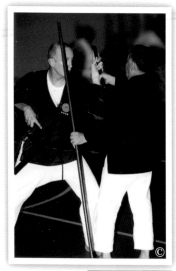

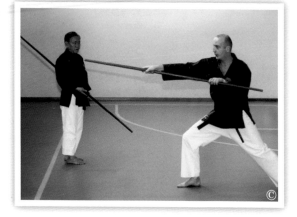

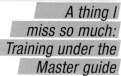

*A thing I miss so much: Training under the Master guide*

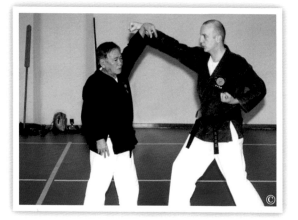

又吉古武道之歷史

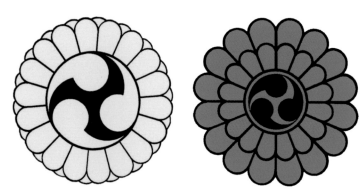

*Old and new brand of the Matayoshi Kobudo.*

The technical background of *Matayoshi Kobudō* is always slowly evolving. Here I present the program of the style of the mid-1990s, when Shinpō Matayoshi died—a snapshot of how it was in that period such as it was taught in *Kōdōkan dōjō*, because in that period there already were differences between *dōjōs* and *Zen Okinawan Kobudō Renmei*. That period, in my opinion, represents the top of the school development. After master Matayoshi's death, the style fragmented into many groups, which were closed to each other and the technical communication stopped.

Furthermore, it is interesting to notice the differences in the teaching program, between what Matayoshi family published two years after the master's death and what really was taught at *Kōdōkan dōjō* before his death: a part of the weapons and their *kata* described have never been witnessed by his older students, not even by *Yoshiaki Gakiya*.

At the end of his life, his older students asserted that there were many things he hadn't transmitted yet and some of the weapons indicated in the list were quite unknown in Okinawa. However the technical program of the ZOKR was set in the 1970s and that of *Kōdōkan* was gradually revised until the 1990s.

47

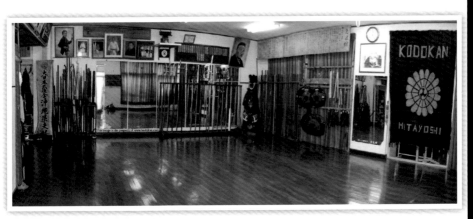

*Kōdōkan Honbu Dōjō*

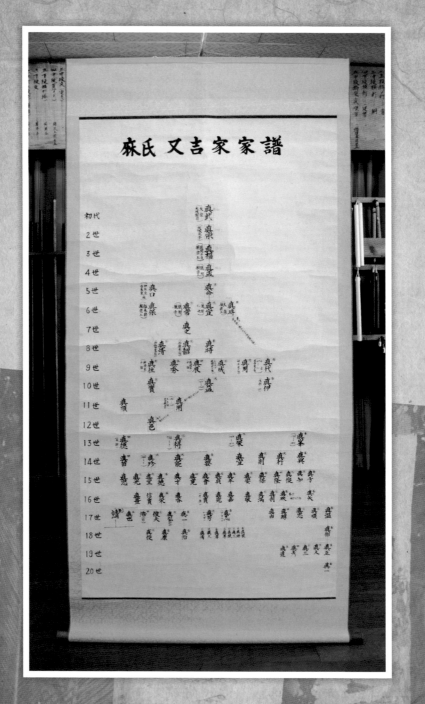

The makimono is a scroll where the family tree is written—This is the family tree of the clan Má relating to the Matayoshi family. The first above is the founder Ufugushiku Shinbu. Then there are many masters and the Sōke of the Matayoshi family among his relatives: thirteenth Shinchin, fourteenth Shintoku, 15th Shinkō, 16th Shinpō, 17th Shinsei (Yasushi).

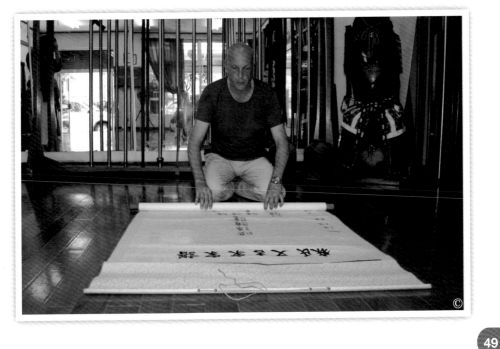

又吉古武道之歴史

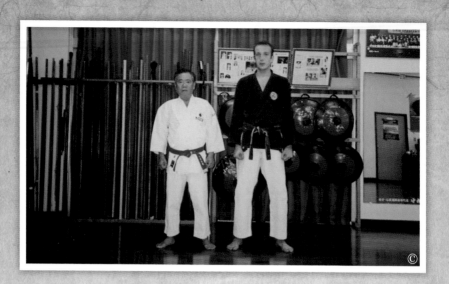

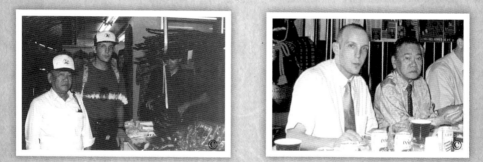

*Some photos of the author with Shinpō Matayoshi Sensei.*

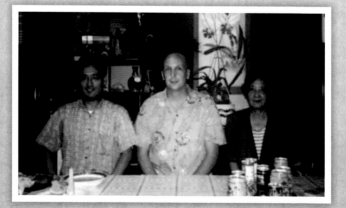

*The author with master Matayoshi's wife and son.*

# Conclusions

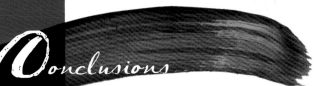

I have had the good fortune and honor to have known Shinpō Sensei and to receive his teaching, to earn his appreciation for my diligence.

My many journeys to Okinawa, my time and resources spent pursuing my passion for Matayoshi Kobudō have been paid back tenfold with his friendship: an honor so rare for a European boy. Now, his memory fills my heart and gives me a sense of my path to being a teacher. Even if nostalgia often prevails, each time I teach something or correct a technique I feel as if he is watching, transmitting his knowledge even now.

I hope it will remain so for future generations: I think the master lived most of all for this reason.

*Shinpō Matayoshi in Italy.*
*A great Master one with:*
*competence, humility, and appeal.*

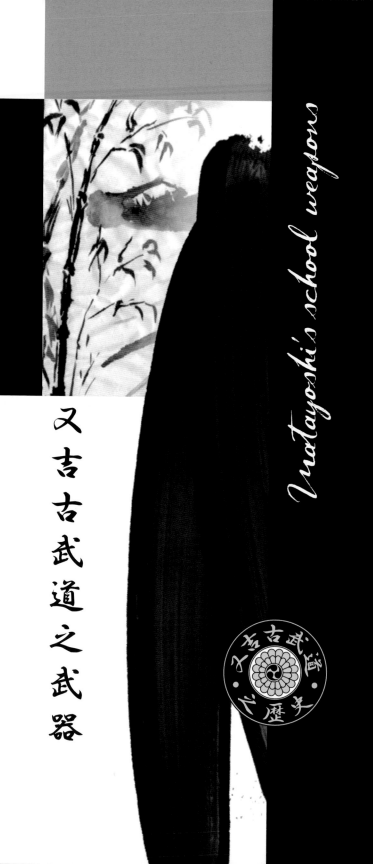

又吉古武道之武器

*Matayoshi's school weapons*

# Introduction

Self-defense arts of *Okinawa* include both combat techniques with and without traditional tools and weapons. Even if weapon techniques represent an important tradition, their future remains uncertain. Modern culture discourages the study of classic weapons for many reasons. First of all, the development of firearms made possible the thinking that the mastery of traditional weapons was obsolete. Moreover there are only a few masters who are experts in wielding these weapons. Finally, to become experts in every self-defense art takes a lot of time, patience, and practice. Today, few people seem to be inclined to to put in the time and effort to learn *Kobudō* deeply.

The study of *Kobudō*, just like that of *Karatedō*, has a value that goes beyond simple physical benefits. It has an historical and cultural value: this discipline has been evolving for centuries and it represents an exceptional progress of human culture. Making perfect *Kobudō* requires an intense and constant physical training that develops with the practice of total control of the body, together with an improvement of strength and a general wellness—all of this combined provides a great benefit to a person's well-being. Of course, we must also consider the self-defense aspect, which is the primary purpose for which *Kobudō* was born. The most important values, which are acquired through *Kobudō* practice are the moral values. The practice teaches humility, respect, loyalty, perseverance, and pride. With scrupulousness and passion the *Kobudō* student strengthens their inner self, building a strong self-esteem.

Most new *Kobudō* practitioners are impressed by the great variety of weapons involved, and by the fact that the evolution of most of them has taken place out of the Ryūkyū archipelago. I hope that this book will bring to light some obscure and little known aspects.

In ancient times, the weapon expert had to master at least three types of weapons. First, they had to have a main weapon, such as a stick or a lance, in which they were the most experienced; this weapon was visible to the rival and it was the most effective. A second weapon had to be hidden on their person, it was possibly a flexible weapon, for use in case of the main weapon had been lost. Then, for long distance use or in case of a surprise attack, they needed a throwing weapon; some of which were easy to hide.

When choosing weapons, these experts had to consider three factors:

1) What type was more suitable for their physical characteristics, especially height and strength

2) Conditions and location of the fight (village, beach, hill, etc.).

3) Their style of handling and their technical preferences.

又吉古武道之歴史

To be able to efficiently use various weapons on different occasions, an expert should practice at least a weapon for each type: long, short, limber, and double. Because the same principles underline the different weapons, it should be easy for a well-trained practitioner to use each weapon immediately. Moreover, they should be able to transform every object within reach into an efficient self-defense tool.

Training with a long weapon used to traditionally start with a long stick (*roku-shaku-bō*). There's even an old saying which goes, "the *roku-shaku-bō* is the root of all long weapons."

Masters affirm that in the first phase of the study it is the man that moves the weapon, in the second phase man and weapon become one, and finally, when perfection is reached, the weapon acquires a soul and a life of its own—the weapon moves the man rather than the other way around.

Moreover, combat strategy determines the weapon that is used. There are many examples of weapons that have been created especially for new self-defense. It is said, for example, that the stick with more sections was created to be used against an enemy with a shield.

又吉古武道之武器

# Weapons of the Matayoshi School

Cataloguing weapons used by Matayoshi Kobudō School can be done using various criteria: length, origin, materials, etc. The categorization used here (long weapons, short, limber, and double) is it not necessarily the most precise–some of these weapons could fall under other categories. The method used here, in any case, should be useful to the passionate people of this discipline.

Some of the weapons are very different from each other because of many factors: place of origin, aim of use, characteristics of the users, etc. An expert *Kobudōka* has to know not only the different weapons, but also to understand the differences between them.

In the century-long history of *Kobudō*, the style, shape, material and productive techniques of the various weapons have been changed countless times.

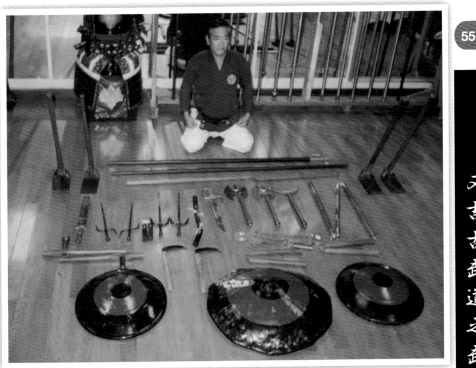

*Kōdōkan Dōjō: Shinpō Matayoshi Sensei*

又吉古武道之武器

Long weapons

又吉古武道之武器

長武器

又吉古武道
之歴史

# Long weapons

Originally there were no defined schemes for weapon making. The weapons were built to suit the individual's needs, taking into account his physical characteristics and his combat style. If the person was tall and strong, a long and heavy weapon was not a problem, but if he wasn't very strong, a shorter and lighter weapon was better.

A long weapon has two advantages over a short one:

1) It has a higher potential efficacy, thanks to its length and to the width of its trajectory

2) Its range of action is wider and it permits to the user to hit first, while keeping a safe distance.

However, there are also some disadvantages: it is more difficult to transport and to conceal them, and if the rival is able "to close the distance," the long weapon loses most of its efficacy.

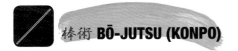

## 棒術 BŌ-JUTSU (KONPO)

### GENERAL INFORMATION

Chinese sources put the birth of the weapon *Gun* (*Kun*) in the last period of the Huang Di dynasty (2690-2590 B.C.). It used to be made of strong wood (birch or oak, for example), which was often dipped in a special oil to improve the resistance at impact. Occasionally there long sticks made of full or hollow metal were used. The circumference of the stick was such that the forefinger and the thumb of the user would, when grasping it, barely touch. The length of the stick varied depending on whether you were in the north or south of China. In the north it was measured by stretching the arm over the head: the stick, resting on the ground, reached the base of the wrist. While in the south, the stick resting on the ground reached only to the height of the eyebrows and for this reason it was called *QimeiGun* "stick of the eyebrows."

In Okinawa the *bō-jutsu* has been in existence since the *Sanzan-jidai* period (1314-1429). Some sources affirm that the art of *bō*, in Okinawa, was reserved for the officials and the king's functionaries, but probably also for simple citizens—fishermen and farmers used it as a work tool and as a tool for defense. According to the Okinawan language dictionary, *bō* is described as: *"the stick for the transport [of weights, such as baskets] and for the martial art."* So, it's likely that between common citizens there already existed knowledge of quite developed *bō* techniques. Chinese techiniques had a great influence on the technical aspects of *bō* development:

• Through Chinese experts who lived in Okinawa as delegates in charge of keeping diplomacy relations with the island royals.

又吉古武道之武器

- Thanks to the action of masters who were part of the Chinese community which settled in Kume village in 1392

- Thanks to of the influence of Chinese stick art, which was introduced to the island by some travelers who had visited China, or who had been sent there by the king of Okinawa.

- In addition to the Chinese influence, some Japanese martial techniques were introduced on the island after the Satsuma invasion in 1609.

The influence of the Chinese invasion has been substantial, and for this reason, many current Okinawan techniques appear to exist in the ancient manuals of Chinese martial arts. A part of the Chinese *Bubishi* (*Wu Bei Zhi*) is titled *Shaolin Konpo* detailing the *Shaolin* stick method reads: "All martial weapons have originated from the stick art, which has originated in the temple of Shaolin." Another ancient Chinese manual (the *Kikoshinsho*) notes "using bō is like reading *The Four Books* and *The Six Theories*" (classical Chinese books), meaning that after you have studied the bō art, it will be easier to learn about other martial arts.

However, *Okinawan bō* is a technique that comes from both Chinese schools and ancient local techniques (*son- bō*) which are then applied to the Okinawan population's body type and to the particular climate and geographical situation on the island.

The *bō* is the main weapon of *Okinawan Kobudō*. On the island it is called *Kon*, which is similar to the Chinese word (*K'un*), demonstrating the strong cultural influence that China has had over Okinawan people. The *bō* art is called *Konpo* (stick method) or *bō-jutsu*. The material used is red or white oak, Japanese plum, areca and "*kuba*" (a sort of palm), which are stout and flexible trees originating in the subtropical zone that includes Okinawa. Most of the *kuba (aukuba)* feature waved venations that it make it difficult to damage it. If broken, the two pieces are lance-sharp and this is one of the many characteristics which make it a perfect wood for *bō* making.

*Okinawan bō* differs in many ways from the Japanese weapon; in fact, they are different in length (excluding the *rokushaku-bō*), shape, use, and most of all grasping. Below we examine some distinctive features of this weapon:

**Division for length:**

The standard length of *Okinawan bō* is 181.8cm. In this case we are referring to the *rokushaku- bō* (a stick six *shaku* long: 1 *shaku* = 30.3cm). In addition to this version which is the most common, there are others that have a length from four *shaku* (*yonshaku- bō*) to a maximum of twelve

58

又吉古武道之武器

shaku ( *junishaku- bō*). There is also a type of *bō* thirteen *shaku* long, called also *bajo- bō* or horse *bō*.

### Division for shape:

The first stick was likely cylindrical (*maru-bō*) and it probably was a *Tenbin*—a stick for transporting heavy loads, carried on the shoulders in the Chinese way. It was likely made of bamboo (*take- bō*). Through the years new shapes and sections have developed. During fighting, sticks with a squared section (*kaku- bō*), hexagonal (*rokkaku- bō*), or octagonal (*hakkaku- bō*) have also been used. These angular *bō* have devastating effects. The shape commonly found today is again the rounded one, but with a biconical section. The stick center (*chukon-bu*) measures 1 *sun* (3.03cm), while the two ends (*kontei*) measures both 8 *bu* (2.424cm). In this way the gravity center of the weapon is perfectly located and handling becomes easier with maximum efficacy. Furthermore, the biconical shape permits the *bō* to wriggle in case of a block by a short or chain weapon. This particular shape gives the *bō* a better resistance against impact and it reduces the risk of breakage.

Take note that *Okinawan Kobudō* also includes some weapons that have base handling in common with the *bō*. These weapons, which we will illustrate later on, are: the *ēku* (*sunakake-bō* or *kai*), the *nunti-bō*, and the *chōgama*. These four weapons must be studied separately.

### SCHOOL PROGRAM

The *bō* is the fundamental weapon of the style—it gives the base for the other weapons, most of all the long weapons and it has the widest technical background. This background is made of: fundamentals, *kata*, and exercises in pairs. The *katas* of this weapon are also in the other weapons school of Okinawa, although often with names and techniques that are very different. This fact recalls the stylistic differences between the same *kata* in *karatedō* in the different schools: *Passai*, *Sanchin*, *Sēsan*, etc. These differences are unavoidable if we consider the limited dimensions of the Okinawan island, which increased the possibility of contact between various teachers of each epoca.

The didactical program of the *Matayoshi* style includes these techniques:

*Hojoundō (bō-jutsukihonwaza)*: in Japanese *hojo* 補助 means "to help" and *undo* 運動 "movement". So the term *hojoundō* indicates the entirety of the movements that help the learning of the base techniques. The *bō* study includes three progressive *hojoundō* made of five sequences of one or more technique: six single techniques and nine combinations.

又吉古武道之武器

These *hojoundō* were created in 1970 by master Shinpō Matayoshi when, at the founding of the *Ryūkyū Kobudō Renmei*, he decided to systemize the teaching program and the rank passages. With the help of his more valuable students and extrapolating the techniques from the *katas*, he composed the *hojoundō* of *bō*, *sai*, *tunkuwa*, and *nunchaku*.

Techniques have to be repeated alternating right and left, going ahead and going back.

<u>*Shushi No Kon*</u>: it is said that this kata has been created by Shushi no Tanmei (old Shushi), a Chinese man who originally came from Shanghai, and who around the mid-1800s went to Okinawa and stayed there. He lived for many years in Naha, in the Azato district, near the Sogen temple. Shushi no Tanmei was a *bō-jutsu* and Chinese Kenpo expert. He taught this stick kata, which was named for him after his death. This traditional *kata*, which is the first to be taught in our school, is one of the most known and practiced by the *kobudōka* of the various schools of Okinawa.

<u>*Choun No Kon*:</u>
CHO = morning
UN = cloud
NO = of
KON = stick.

Meaning: "stick of the morning cloud." This kata was created around 250 years ago by a warrior of *Tomari*, who was known as *Choun Oyakata* from which it takes the name. *Choun* taught his kata to many people, which became popular through the *bujin*, most of all in *Tomari*, where it was considered very valuable because of its frequent changes of direction.

<u>Sakugawa No Kon (Chinen Yamani-no Kon):</u> Chinen Chikudun Peichin Umikana, nicknamed "Aburayayamashiro" (1797-1881), developed this kata after some research about ancient *bō* techniques in the villages (*sonbō*). The kata takes the name from *Sakugawa Kanga* (*Teruya Chikudun Pēchin Kanga*), master of *Chinen Umikana*. Some theories support that this form has been handed down directly by Sakugawa. Shinkō Matayoshi who learned this *kata* from Sanra Chinen (Chinen Yamani - 1842-1925), Umikana's son.

<u>Chikin No Kon:</u> this *kata*, called also Chikin-bo or Ken-ka-Bo, was transmitted by Chikin Seisoku (Shosoku) Oyakata and it was

又吉古武道之武器

composed by some fishermen of the Shoren village on Tsuken Island. It contains counterattacks (*gyakuwaza*), and techniques to fight against a lance. Matayoshi Shinkō learned it from Chokuho Agena.

Shiishi No Kon (Soeishi no kon in Japanese): it is taught that this kata is more than 300 years old and that it was created by Oyakata Shiishi, a noble instructor of martial arts in the Ryūkyū reign. For many years it was transmitted only through first born sons of the Shiishi family and the Ryūkyū royal family. Shinkō Matayoshi learned it from a Shiishi's family descendant, Ryuko Shiishi.

In Okinawa, after learning the *hojoundō*, Matayoshi Kobudō students learn the kata *Shushi no kon*. However, many advanced students of master *Matayoshi*, thinking that this kata is too difficult for a beginner, have created some base *kata*. The author has created a base kata for this weapon, called *Bō kihon kata*, based on the techniques of the first and second *hojoundō*. He also created a base *kata* for elementary school children: *Bō kiso kata*.

Kumiwaza and Oyo: in pairs or in groups of three (a tori and two uke), the applications of the techniques of *Shushi no kon* and *Choun no kon* are trained quite regularly in the *Kōdōkan*

*dōjō* but rarely that of the other *kata*.

There are also some *bō* sequences against other weapons, using different techniques of the kata, which have been developed by some of master Matayoshi's students. They are sequences of different lengths: from the entire form of the kata to the single technique application.

Except for the *hojoundō*, the techniques in pairs are trained in a more free way against the *kata*. However, there are some fixed rules to easily develop each technique. This system of application is one of the stronger points of the school.

*Shinpō Matayoshi* created a base *Kumibō* (application of the first *bō hojoundo*). The author has developed other two *Kumibō*, based on the second and third *hojoundō*. Other students of Shinpō Matayoshi also developed some *Kumibō*.

Analyzing the *Matayoshi Kobudō* history we can observe that in the field of this school other kata of *bō* have been studied (but which are no longer studied): *Kubo no kon* (from the name of the *Kubo* area, in the *Gushikawa* village), *Yuniga* or *Yonegawa no kon* (from the name of the *Yonegawa* area, in the *Shuri* distict), *Yara no kon* (a variation of *ChatanYara no kon*), all taught by *Shinchin Matayoshi. Shinkō Matayoshi* learned *Ufugushiku* (*Oshiro*) *no Kon* from *Chojo Oshiro*, while *Shinpō*

又吉古武道之武器

*Matayoshi* learned *Tokumine no kon* from *Chotoku Kyan*.

Moreover, some of *Shinpō's* expert students also practiced *Ufuton no kon* (*Ufuton-bō*), which they learned from a local teacher, on master's invitation. Shusei Maeshiro together with some other older students, went to teacher of *Uechi-ryū* to learn this kata, which was later adapted to the characteristics of the *Matayoshi* School.

When codifying his teaching system Shinpō Matayoshi chose to teach only five main kata, although students decided to preserve additional kata. When Shinpō Matayoshi died, only the five main kata were considered part of the official style.

The *Matayoshi* style include also techniques for eight or nine *shaku bō*, which are occasionally demonstrated using *Sakugawa no kon*, even if this *kata* doesn't represent all the various techniques for a long weapon. In the *Junshinka dōjō*, the author's students practice these kata: *Shushi*, *Choun*, *Sakugawa*, *Chikin*, *Shiishi*. *Ufuton*, *Tokumine*, *Yuniga*, *Kubo*, *Oshiro* and *Yara* are taught also to the *uchi-deshi* to preserve the whole technical background.

## GENERAL INFORMATION

This technique developed in Ryūkyū thanks to a fisherman of Tsuken-jima called Akachu (red man) because of his complexion due to the suntan he got at sea. Master Chikin Shosoku Oyakata was condemned to death for fighting for power in the Shuri town. He was greatly respected because he was a *bō-jutsu* expert. Because of this expertise, rather than face execution, he was exiled to the island of *Tsuken-jima* where he lived with an unpretentious fisherman named Akachu, but who was called Azato. Chikin decided to teach Azato the *bō* art and soon the student, who was very proficient, exceeded the master. After learning the techniques of the master, Azato created an oar *kata* for self-defense against enemies with sword, lance, or stick. He modified his oar so the blade edge (*name-giri*) was so sharp as to cut flesh.

The oar is a very powerful and efficient weapon for attack and defense techniques using each part of the tool. One of the most particular and valuable techniques is called *sunakake* (to throw sand). The oar, which is also called *ryoshi no Katana* (fishermen sword), is also practiced in some places in China, where it is called *"zhao."*

## SCHOOL PROGRAM

*Ēku* techniques of *Matayoshi* style come from two sources: the *Matayoshi* family, in which tradition said it was *Shinchin Matayoshi's* favorite weapon, and *Agena Chokuho*. The *kata* is called *Chikin Akachu no ēkudi,* "techniques of the red man from *Chikin (Tsuken)*" in memory of its creator.

*Shinpō Matayoshi* considered this his favorite weapon, and he always demonstrated *Ēku* in public. The original oar of the *Matayoshi* family, as per master *Shinpō's* will, was cremated with the master's body in September 1997.

To help students learn of the *ōku* fundamentals, the author has created a *hojoundō* of eight sequences.

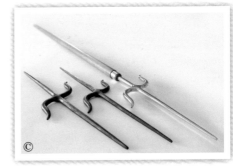 貫手術 **NUNTI-JUTSU (Nunti and Nuntibō)**

### GENERAL INFORMATION

*Nunti* means "perforating weapons." In China there is a manual called *"WubeiZhi,"* that in Japanese is *Bubishi*, (not to be confused with the Okinawa treatise by the same name), that is the "Treatise about the military equipment" written in 1621 by *Mao Yuanyi* (1594-1640), who was a navy official at the time of the *Ming* dynasty. It is the most complete martial arts manual of the Chinese history; it speaks about this weapon, which is called *"saibu* 又武*."* In the book it is affirmed that this weapon was born during the Ming dynasty epoch.

The *nunti*, which resembles a lance point, was introduced in Okinawa from China, together with other weapons, around 600 years ago. Master *Shinkō Matayoshi* learned the *nunti-jutsu* art from an old Chinese master *Jin Ying (Kingai)* in *Shangai (Cina)*.

The *nunti*, put on a five *shaku bō* (150cm about) makes a weapon called *nunti- bō*. A similar tool was used by fishermen as a harpoon. The *Nunti- bō* techniques are very similar to *bō* techniques which originated in the *Tsuken* island, in the *Ryūkyū* archipelago. Using *nunti- bō* as a weapon, you can bring two *nunti* threaded in the belt, both on the abdomen and back. These *nunti* can be thrown against a rival.

又吉古武道之武器

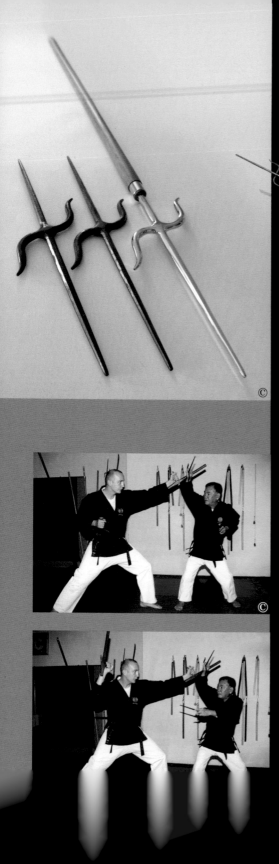

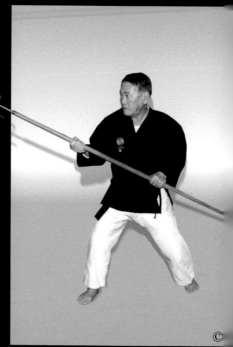

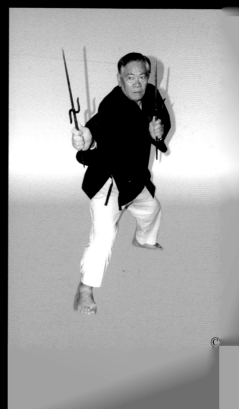

## SCHOOL PROGRAM

The *nunti* are normally used as hand-held weapons, even if they can be used as well as *manji-sai*, which are used as throwing weapons. The throwing weapons, similar to that of the *sai*, are included in the *kata* and they target the feet, even if in reality they can be aimed at each body part. There is only one *kata* for this weapon: *Nunti-bō no kata* (*Nunti no ti*). However, in some demonstrations, there are variations of this *kata* and some of master *Matayoshi's* students have started the study of this weapon executing the *bō kata Chikin no kon*, adapted to the *nunti-bō* techniques.

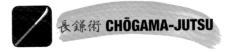

長鎌術 **CHŌGAMA-JUTSU**

### GENERAL INFORMATION

*Chōgama* means "long scythe" and it consists of a half-moon blade put on a long stick of around four *shaku*. This weapon of mixed origin, from both war and agricultural purposes, has a total length of about 170 cm. It takes from *bō* some base movement widened with cutting ability. The *chōgama* has a similar shape to the Japanese *naginata*, but it is shorter and its blade is a little bit longer.

There is also a long scythe with a similar blade to that of the *nichōgama*,

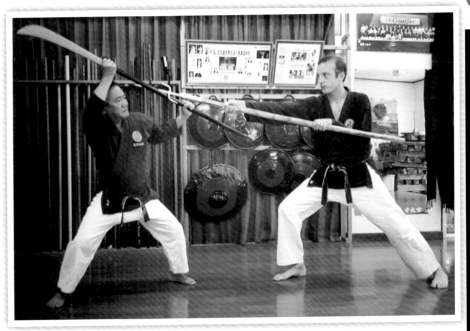

*Kōdōkan Dōjō: Shinpō Matayoshi Sensei (chōgama) and the author (nuntibō)*

又吉古武道之武器

that is, perpendicular to the wooden handle, it is the *rokusahku-gama* (six foot-long scythe).

There is then a variant used by the master *Matayoshi*, the *Toyeinoborika-ma*. This weapon has the same characteristics of the *chōgama* but its blade is more curved like a hook. The blade hooks up the body or the weapon of the rival for then hitting him with the wooden part.

### SCHOOL PROGRAM

The handling of this weapon has been shown only to a few students of the school. There isn't a *kata* of *chōgama* but only a series of exercises to practice individually or in pairs. On some occasions, these individual exercises have been composed to form a demonstrative *kata*.

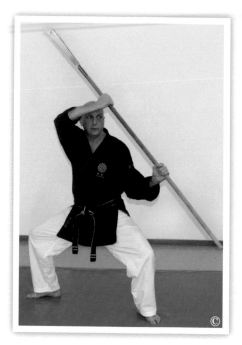

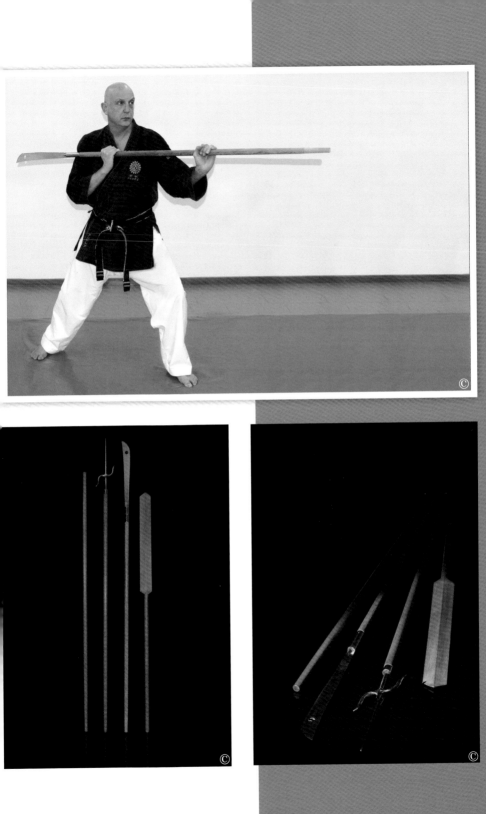

又吉古武道之武器

短武器

*Short weapons*

# Short weapons

The short weapons can have varying lengths, moreover they have a great advantage over the longs: they are easier to transport. Because of their shorter range of action they are used more often for defense than attack. Also limber weapons such as the *nunchaku*, and double weapons such as *sai*, *tunkuwa*, *kama*, *tekko* and *tecchyu*, can be listed in this type of weapon, thought I prefer to discuss them separately.

## 杖術 JŌ-JUTSU (TSUE)

### GENERAL INFORMATION

The *jō* has a length of 127.56 cm (four *shaku*, two *sun*, one *bu*), with a diameter of 24.24 mm (eight *bu*). There are numerous stories about the origin of this tool; this is most of all due to the fact that it is a very simple and diverse weapon of different shapes and lengths. One of the most reliable versions is that the *jō* was simply a walking-stick transformed in an efficient tool of self-defense in case of need. Its length varies in relation to the user height; so there are *jō* which vary from three (*gusan*) to four *shaku*.

©

## SCHOOL PROGRAM

In some *Okinawan dōjō* and in the A.I-K.O. organization, we theach a *jō* form which has been developed by a student of master *Shinpō Matayoshi*, *Kanei Katsuyoshi*, after he studied *Shindo Muso-ryujōdō* with the encouragement of the master himself. This form, called *Jō-jutsu no kata* (杖術之型), studies different techniques of defense and attack, grasping the *jō* quite like a sword.

## 鍬術 KUWA-JUTSU (KUE)

### GENERAL INFORMATION

The origin of this art is similar to that of the *kama*; in fact it is a technique developed by the agricultural or countrymen class. For attack techniques: blade edge, blade head, and handle point are used. A technique which is often used in the *kata* includes throwing dirt in the rival's eyes then to hit him quickly with the *kuwa*. The technique of this weapon is even more refined thanks to the meeting of the countrymen with some *Okinawan* martial arts masters and some Chinese experts. The prototype of this tool differed from the present shape because its handle, even if it had a metal blade, was fixed with an animal horn or a stone. The handle is about three *shaku* (90.3) and it is inserted in a blade at angle between 45 and 60°. There are four

又吉古武道之武器

types of blades: *hiragwe* with a single rectangular blade (used by the *Matayoshi* School), *ishigwe* that is similar to the first but with a stone blade, *tamtaa* which is a bifurcate blade and *mimataa* with a trifurcate blade.

Also now there are some experts of the Chinese *kuwa (chutou)* in *Fuzhou* and *Shangai* (China). Some Chinese experts believe that the use of the hoe as self-defense weapon in the country uprising comes from the *Shen Nong* emperor epoch (237 B.C.), during the era of the "combat states". Often, in China was used a type of hoe (*Ba Tou*) which handle was as long as *bō*; this weapon is nowadays used in some styles of the South such as the *Hung Gar*.

### SCHOOL PROGRAM

In Okinawa the *kuwa*, an agricultural hoe, is only in the *Matayoshi Kobudō* School.

The *Kuwa nu ti kata* (hoe techniques), in the opinion of some old students of *Shinpō Matayoshi*, were created by the master, inspired by techniques which had been passed to his family, even if in some sequences there are clear Chinese influences.

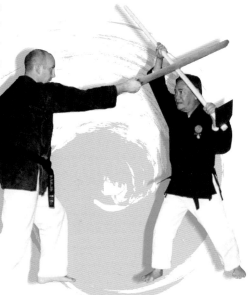

*Shinpō Matayoshi Sensei (kuwa) and the author (ēku)*

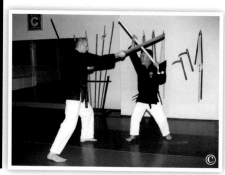

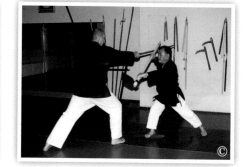

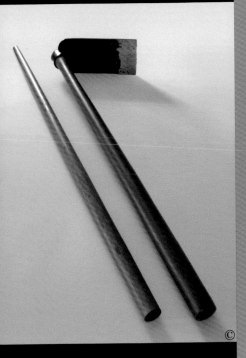

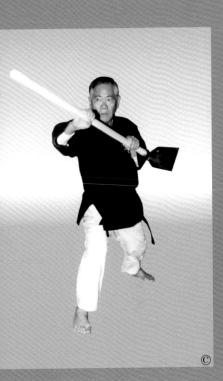

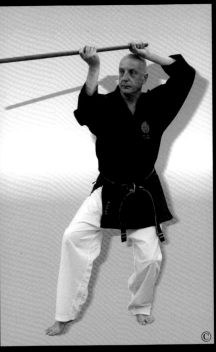

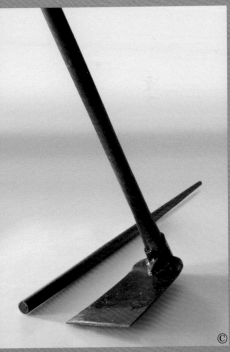

又吉古武道之武器

柔軟武器

*Short weapons*

# *Soft weapons*

The so called "soft" weapons comprise both folding and limber weapons. Their length varies greatly from as short as thirty cm to as long as nine m. These types of tools were normally secondary weapons, to use after the main weapons and they could be easily hidden: around the waist on a belt(*suruchin*), in the sleeves (*nunchaku*) or on the back (*sansetsukon*), without creating obstacles during a fight.

## 双節棍術
## NUNCHAKU-JUTSU
## (Sōsetsukon)

### GENERAL INFORMATION

It is said that after the invasion of the *Ryūkyū* Islands by the *Shimazu* clan, the *nunchaku* was adapted from and inspired by an agricultural tool, as a self-defense tool for women. Another theory states that the *nunchaku* is the derivation of the bit used for horses (*mugenunchaku*). Yet another hypothesis says that some migrants from China, starting from the XII century, knew the use of this tool and that the Okinawan people, who joined the Chinese community of the village of *Kume*, learned how to use it. It is certain, in any case, that the same weapon (*shuang-chiehkun*, *saotsekun*), was used in China many centuries before (around 960 B.C.). It was made of two rounded bars united with a metal chain.

The *nunchaku* of Okinawa consists of two wood octagonal sticks with a cylindrical shape united together with a cord or horsehair. The length of the sticks differs to suit the physical characteristics of the users. The ancient *nunchaku* was a little bit shorter than the present; it was hidden under the clothes for self-defense. Finally, there are *nunchaku* models of three or four sections.

The *nunchaku* is difficult to block because of his flexibility and its ability, to bounce off the target and to hit repeatedly.

### SCHOOL PROGRAM

The *nunchaku* techniques also come from *Okina Irei*. The pronunciation of characters (that it has to be read "*sōsetsukon*" or stick of two sections) is supposed to have come from *Fujian*. There is a *hojoundō* of eight techniques codified in the *Kōdōkan dōjō*, but it is rarely practiced, while the one of ten techniques elaborated by the author is trained in many countries. The author of this book has developed also a second *kata* of *nunchaku* (*Nunchaku dai ni*) and a base *kata*:

©

73

又吉古武道之武器

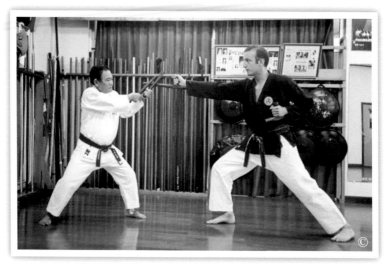

*Kōdōkan Dōjō: Shinpō Matayoshi Sensei (nunchaku) and the author (tunkuwa)*

*Nunchaku kiso kata.* The *Matayoshi no nunchaku kata* is sometimes called as *Nunchaku dai san.* In all likelihood, it was taught, with minimum variations, in the 1960s.

The *nunchaku* with three sections (a small *sansetsukon*) is sometimes used in the *dōjō* but, while the other forms have their own techniques, for this variant of the weapon there is no traditional *kata.* For this reason the author has created a *kata*, called *Sanbon nunchaku.* He has also developed two pre-arranged fighting of *nunchaku* vs *bō: Nunchaku kihon kumite nchaku renzoku kumite.*

### 三節棍術
### SANSETSUKON-JUT-SU

## GENERAL INFORMATION

This is an ancient Chinese weapon that is described in the local writings as "*San-chieh-kun* of the *Shaolin* temple." It is made of three sticks, which are about 70 cm long, joined with a cord or chain. The ends which are not joined with a chain can be covered by metal plug to protect the wood in case of impact—for this reason it is a very long and a more advantageous weapon than others. The main movements are circular, like a fishing reel, or it can be used like a stick or *issetsu* (one section), or *nissetsu* (two sections) or *sansetsu* (three sections). The *sansetsukon* is considered as the "big brother" of the *nunchaku.* A legend says that the inventor of this weapon was the *Jin Hong Yan* general, first em-

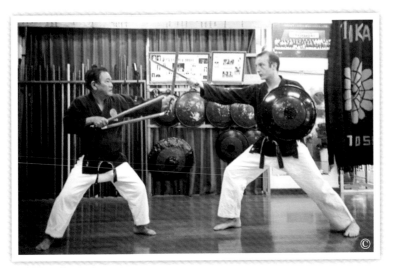

*Kōdōkan Dōjō: Shinpō Matayoshi Sensei (sansetsukon) and the author (tinbē)*

peror of the *Song* Chinese dynasty (960-1279). Also developed in China is a shorter *sansetsukon*, created to be easily transported and hidden. In the *Matayoshi* School the central stick, cylindrical, is a little bit shorter than the extremities (a little bit conical). There is also a limber stick of four short sections (*yonsetsukon*).

### SCHOOL PROGRAM

The *Matayoshi* School is the only style of *Okinawan Kobudō* that teaches the use of this weapon. There is only a classical *kata*, which was perhaps created by *Shinpō Matayoshi* based on the movements his father taught to him. This long and complex *kata* called *Sansetsukon nu ti* has never been shown in public. Only a few students of master *Matayoshi*, including *Yoshiaki Gakiya* and the author, know this *kata* correctly.

A second shorter *kata*, called *Hakuho* (白鵬), was developed by *Shinpō Matayoshi*'s student, and it has been taught widely since the 1980s. This *kata*, which

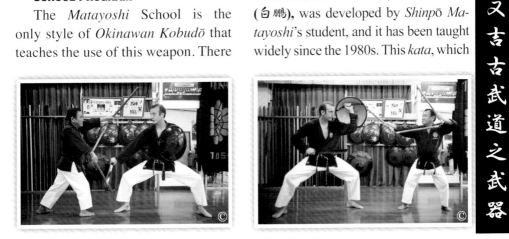

又吉古武道之武器

is extremely valuable for the didactical point of view, is often shown in public. Because it is the simplest classical *kata*, it is taught as first and it is called *Sansetsukon dai ichi;* in this case, the other *kata* is called *Sansetsukon dai ni.*

A student of master *Matayoshi* has created two *hojoundō* of five techniques and they have been reviewed by the author. The practice of these two *hojoundō* is essential to acquire a solid base of movements with the *sansetsukon.*

双流星術
## SURUCHIN-JUTSU

### GENERAL INFORMATION

The *suruchin* origin dates back to the Stone Age where it was used as a defense tool against wild animals. Originally it was built with a cord made by the bark called *surukaa* from which the name is derived. The *suruchin* technique consists of rotating the weapon with the aim to hit or to hook up the rival's limbs or neck. This weapon existed in Okinawa for a long period, but it has been spread widely with the introduction on the ancient techniques of the Chinese lash (*biân*).

The *suruchin* can have different lengths: three *shaku* (90.9 cm), five *shaku* (151.5 cm), six *shaku* (181.8 cm), eight *shaku* (242.4 cm). The shorter *suruchin* are often used to hit, with the aim to get tangled in the rival's body or to unhorse him. The standard size, used in the *Matayoshi* School, is proportionate to the user. A similar weapon to the *suruchin* can be found in every part of the world, where they have been developed for self-defense reasons, to hunt or to catch the animals destined for breeding (for example the Argentinian bolas). In ancient times, some experts wore it as a belt.

The *suruchin* of the *Matayoshi* School is made of a cord that puts together two holed stones. The holes permit affixing the stones with the cord with strength. However, there are, in more recent years, some forms of this weapon in which the cord has been replaced with a chain.

It is useful to remember that in the past master *Shinpō Matayoshi* taught also the single stone *suruchin.* The techniques come from the master *Kingai*, but we suppose that they have also been influenced by the *Ryūkyū Kobudō* techniques.

*Shinpō Matayoshi* was a great expert in using *suruchin* and he could entrap an enemy's weapon, disarming him with apparent ease. He also demonstrated blocking techniques against a weapon taking it tight with the *suruchin*, grasping the other end quickly in order to attack the enemy's vital points.

In 1880, the *Nanto Zatsuwa* magazine published an illustration showing the use of the *suruchin:* in Naha, two well-dressed children of *Satsuma*, with the *tanto* (knife) on their belt, were practicing some techniques, both against each other, with a rounded stone tied up to a cord, while other Okinawa children, modestly dressed, were watching them.

In the end there are some *suruchin* composed of a chain with two metal weights on the ends. Some people think that this type of weapon comes from a tool to measure weight, used by merchants and dealers of Okinawa.

### SCHOOL PROGRAM

The use of the *suruchin* includes many techniques of rotation (*furi*),

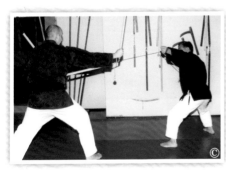

thrusts (*zuki*), defenses (*uke*), grasping changes (*mochikae*), grips (*hikitori*), stop in the air (*furidome*), hooking (*karage*), lengthening (*nobashi*), shortening (*chijime*), etc. Even if many techniques of this weapon are taught and the most expert students use it in many ways during demonstrations and practice, there is not a classical *kata* of *suruchin*.

In Okinawa, on master Ma- tayoshi's recommendation, there is a *kata* of *suruchin* which has often been demonstrated by his student *Kenichi Yamashiro*. This form, called *Suruchin no Toseki* (throwing the stone) has been expanded with more complex techniques by the author and

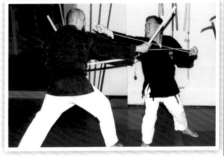

he has also created some *hojoundō* base techniques to the training of this most complex weapon.

車棒術
# KURUMANBŌ-JUTSU

又吉古武道之武器

## GENERAL INFORMATION

It is a five *shaku* long stick on which is fixed, through a pivot wood, to another stick of about fifty cm. It is possible to see some models of this tool and others of *Kobudō* in the Okinawa prefectural museum (in *Naha*).

Originally, the *kurumanbō* was an ancient country tool (scourge) that was used in farming, and it was transformed in a very old art, sister of the *nunchaku* and the *sansetsukon*. In the *Kume* village (Okinawa) there is an old document about the history of this place which mentions this weapon. Some schools call this tool *Renkuwan*.

In China there is a similar weapon called *Shaokun* (sentinels' stick) o *Shaozi*. It is composed of a stick about 160cm long on which is fixed, with a cord or a chain, a shorter stick. This weapon was used to hit the horses' hooves or to fight against enemies with a shield.

It is interesting to highlight that a similar tool is used currently by the farmers in some Italian regions to work legumes and cereals.

## SCHOOL PROGRAM

The *kuruman- bō kata* has been taught by master *Matayoshi* only in his latest years of life. It is a very particular form, and it is one of the few *kata* in our school that contains a kick technique (in this case *mae-geri*).

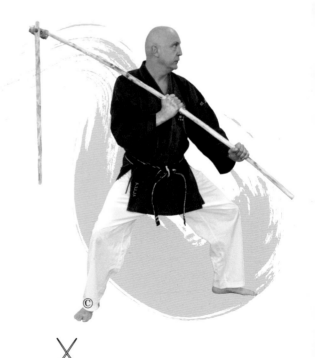

又吉古武道之武器

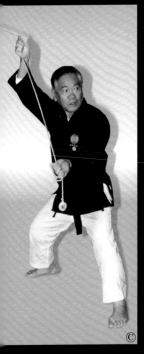

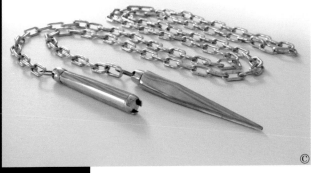

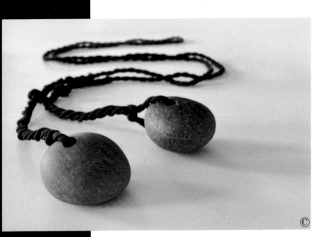

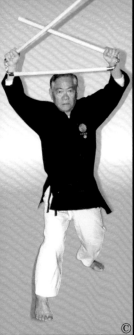

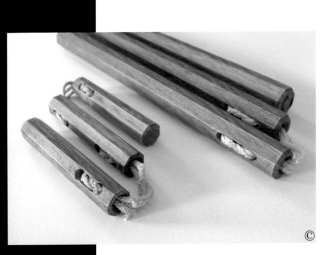

*Double weapons*

又吉古武道之武器

双武器

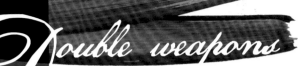

# Double weapons

This type of weapon makes use of different types of materials: wood, metal, bamboo, animal skin, etc. They often are main defense weapons, in which the individual specializes. Some movements of this weapon are similar to each other; after mastering one weapon, it allows one to use another easily. The origins of the various weapons are many: agricultural, fishing, symbolic tools or real actual weapons. Some of these, such as *sai* and *tunkuwa*, are considered base weapons; others as *kama* and *tinbē* are surely advanced weapons while *tekko* and *tecchu* are studied rarely in the *Matayoshi* school and only at a very high level.

## 釵術 SAI-JUTSU

### GENERAL INFORMATION

This metal trident has a long history. We can find similar tools in many countries in Southeast Asia: China (the *T'ieh-ch'ih*), India and Indonesia. It is supposed that some sailors of *Sumatra* or *Java* introduced them in the *Ryūkyū* archipelago. Another theory is that the *sai* had been introduced in Okinawa by Chinese monks who were men of martial arts. The weapons of these monks were simpler and adapted versions for the practical use of some objects we can find in the ancient Chinese and Indian sacred iconography: they are symbols of power made to protect the Buddhist doctrine. The *sai*, for example, seems to have been developed from the form of the Indra's sword, a great Indian God who was incorporated into Buddhism as a protective God.

Another theory suggests that this tool originally was a hairpin, which transformed into a very short weapon similar to a dagger which then became the *sai*. Without knowing its exact origin, it is told that this weapon comes from the Ming dynasty (1368-1644).

In Okinawa, some non-commissioned police officers called "*Chikusaji*" brought and used this self-defense tool which could be thrown against anyone who offered resistance to arrest. The goal of throwing was to knock down the escaping criminal allowing an easy arrest. These throwing techniques are preserved in some *kata*.

Fundamentally the *sai* are used in pairs, one for each hand. In some superior *kata* the *kobudōka* can have an additional third *sai* placed in the belt in front of or back. The third *sai* is useful to

81

又吉古武道之武器

replace the sai that eventually is thrown in the rival's direction.

## SCHOOL PROGRAM

The *sai* techniques taught in the *Matayoshi* style come from those taught to *Shinkō Matayoshi* from *Chokuho Agena*. For this weapon there is a *hojoundō* of ten fundamental techniques, practiced both individually and in pairs. There are three *kata*: *Nichō sai*, *Sanchō sai* and *Shinbaru no sai.* Some practitioners call these *kata*, especially the first two, "*Matayoshi no sai*" but *Shinpō Matayoshi* was very hostile to this custom. *Nichō sai* and *Sanchōsai* were created as forms for training by *Shinpō Matayoshi* after the First World War, while *Shinbaru no sai* has been taught by *Shinkō Matayoshi*. We have to remember that *Shinbaru* is the name of the district, situated in the *Chatan* village, where *Shinkō* grew up. *Shinbaru* (千原), in Japanese "senhara," means "hundred plains".

*Sanchō sai* and *Shinbaru no sai* are executed using three *sai*. In both these *kata* there are two *sai* throwing techniques: after the first *sai* has been thrown, this is immediately replaced by the other, which is on the belt. This is quite difficult to execute in the *dōjō*; for this reason throwing techniques are trained with appropriate targets or outdoors.

The *Matayoshi* style also works with the *Matayoshi-sai*, even if they are something that only some expert students have learned and they are not frequently taught. It is a *sai* variant called *Manji-sai*. While the handle is similar to that of the *sai*, the hilt is like an "s," that is, the same as the *nunti*. The name *Matayoshi-sai (sai of Matayoshi)* originates from the fact that *Shinkō Matayoshi* was the first Okinawa expert to build this tool based on a similar tool he had seen in *Shangai* (China). This type of overturned hilt is in many different weapons of the South China.

There isn't specific *kata* for the *Matayoshi-sai,* so these weapon techniques are the same of the *sai-jutsu*, except for some specific techniques. *Shinbaru no sai kata* is often demonstrated with this particular weapon.

In the *sai-jutsu*, except for the *hojoundō*, working in pairs is less formal and more individualized; for this reason the author has developed two pre-arranged fighting of *sai* vs *bō* (*Sai kihon kumite* and *Sai renzoku kumite*). He has created also a base *kata* for

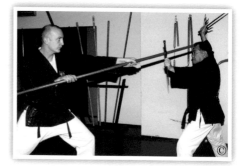

82

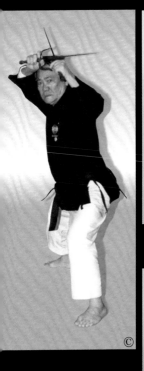

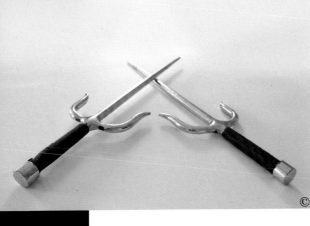

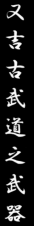

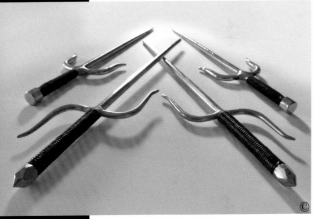

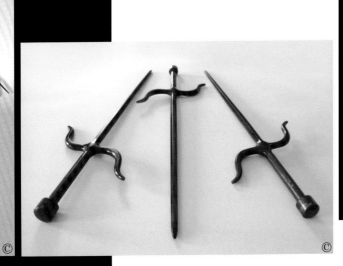

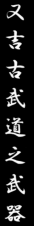

又吉古武道之武器

*Sai kiso kata.*

柱拐術

# TUNKUWA-JUT-SU
# (Tonfa)

## GENERAL INFORMATION

This weapon is called "*Tonfa*," "*Tunfa*," or "*Tuifa*." Inspired by the the handle of a particular grain mortar and other agricultural tools, this improvised weapon has a formidable efficacy in the hand of an expert countryman. The *tunkuwa* is made of wood and it has a length of about fifty cm. At three-quarters of the length there a biconical handle is set perpendicular to the length which permits an efficient use. In case of need, the *tunkuwa* could be rapidly used and it was quite impossible for the enemy to suspect the power of this tool, which appeared harmless.

It is impossible to confirm exactly when the *tunkuwa* was transformed into a weapon; the same tool is traditionally used by numerous populations in the Orient, most of all by the Chinese (some *Kung-Fu* schools teach nowadays some of the *tunkuwa kata*, called *Shuang*

©

*Kuai*). In China (in the province of *Shouxi*) some people think that it was born thanks to the master *Sun Bin*, a military strategist who lived between the "Spring-Autumn period" and the "Fighting Countries" period (722-222 B.C.). In Thailand there exists a tool very similar to the *tunkuwa* that is affixed to the forearm with a little cord. In the *Ryūkyū* its use spread most of all after the abolition of the clans and the institution of the Okinawa prefecture. As has happened for many *Kobudō* weapons, it has been camouflaged as a common-use tool; in this case it was a Chinese millstone, called "*toushi*" in the local dialect.

In Okinawa, in the course of the time, the systematization of the martial use of the *tunkuwa* and the creation of a real method starting from the experience were born at the same time in many villages for self-defense reasons.

The *tunkuwa-jutsu* requires wrist agility and a balanced use of the grip intensity. The speed of the arm movements and the comeback (*osame*) has also an important role, as well as the speed of the grip changing (*mochikae*).

The best wood for the *tunkuwa* construction is the same used for the *bō* and the other wood weapons: oak, red oak and Japanese plum.

In recent decades many mil-

84

又吉古武道之武器

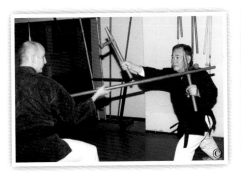 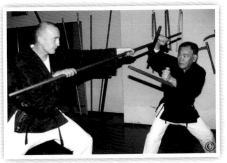

itary corps and police forces have introduced the use of *tunkuwa* into their line of self-defense tools. Strangely, this tool is not used for this aim in Japan nor in the Okinawa prefecture. The *tunkuwa* techniques of the *Matayoshi* School come from master *Irei Okina*.

### SCHOOL PROGRAM

For the study of the *tunkuwa* there is a *hojoundō* of ten fundamental techniques, which is practiced both individually and in pairs. There is also a *hojoundō* with the special grasp (*Tokushu mochi*) created by the author taking inspiration from some techniques which had been shown by master *Matayoshi*.

The program includes the study of two *kata: Tunkuwa dai ichi* and *Tunkuwa dai ni*. There is also a demonstrative *kata: Tunkuwa ni dan* (sometimes called *dai san*), that is very similar to the first and it contains some techniques of the second. Many expert students have contributed with personal variations in the forms

of *tunkuwa* and in creating the base *kata*, but in the *Kōdōkan dōjō* only these three *kata* are taught. The author has created another advanced *kata*, *Tunkuwa dai san*, which is taught in the A.I.K.O program. He has also codified two pre-arranged *tunkuwa* fighting against *bō* (*Tunkuwa kihon kumite* and *Tunkuwa tai bō renzoku kumite*) ase *kata* for children: *Tunkuwa a*.

籐牌術
## TINBĒ-JUTSU
### (Tinbē and bantō/ seiryuto)

### GENERAL INFORMATION

The shield and the armor have always been considered very important in ancient military defense. Particularly the shield exists in all cultures on every continent. The shields were usually rectangular or rounded; normally the rectangular, bigger and heavier, were brought by the infantry. The rounded and light, made of

又吉古武道之武器

Indian cane (*teng-pai*), were used in man-to-man fighting. The Indian cane (rattan) is a very strong and light climbing plant, which grows in South China. The *tinbē-jutsu* is one of the techniques *Shinkō Matayoshi* learned from the old and venerated master *Kingai*. At the time of the conflict between the three reigns of Okinawa (*Sanzan jidai*), the *tinbē* was already used in real fighting.

A shield that can be built in these ways:

• Using the bark of a particular tree called "*bin-lo.*" This bark is worked and treated with a specific oil to model its shape and to make it more resistant.

• Building a rattan frame, or of another wood type, and covering it with an animal skin.

• In metal: with the advancements of the metallurgy it would be possible to create shields in metal, strong but light.

On the shield there was often painted the symbol of the membership school. Another decoration was to draw particular figures to impress the enemies. This shield has to be used with a little sword (*bantō*) and together they make the *tinbē-jutsu* art.

86

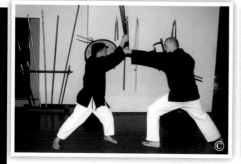

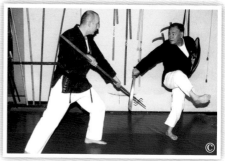

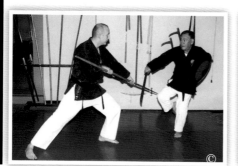

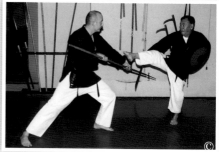

又吉古武道之武器

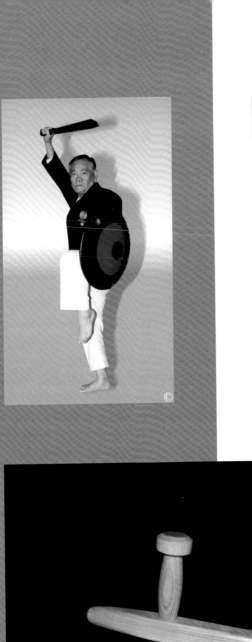

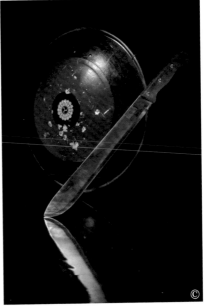

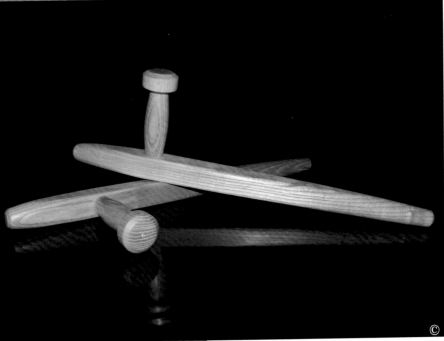

又吉古武道之武器

Some Okinawa schools now use this type of *tinbē* got from the carapace of a sea tortoise and it is used together with a small lance (*rochin*).

## SCHOOL PROGRAM

The metal shield (aluminum) has replaced definitively that of *rattan* and it permits use in pair exercises, without damaging it quickly. I went personally with master *Matayoshi* to the *Hei-wa-dori* market in *Naha* to buy some big lids for woks (Chinese pan) with which to obtain the modern *tinbē*. In *Kōdōkan dōjō* there is also a big *tinbē* with the *rattan* frame covered with a hardened ox skin. *Shinpō Matayoshi* used the *tinbē* also with a little sword with hilt, typical of the South China styles. The *tinbē-jutsu* of the *Matayoshi* School, taught by master *Kingai*, is really called the *tinbē* of the Chinese techniques of the *Kingai* School (*Kingai ryu*). The *kata Tinbē nu ti* or *Matayoshi no tinbē* was composed by *Shinpō Matayoshi* on the basis of the *NICHŌGAMA-JUTSU*. However it is told that this form has been influenced also by *tinbē* techniques of the *Ryūkyū Kobu-jutsu*.

## GENERAL INFORMATION

The use of iron for the agricultural tools in *Okinawan* began around 700 years ago. In the same epoch the first weapons were imported from Japan and China. The scythe was a tool used by farmers to cut hay, canes, and straw; only later it was used as a weapon. Because bandits met often to steal in the villages, it became usual to practice combat techniques with this tool to protect both property and life.

The *kama* was used as a weapon for the first time during a peasant's rebellion in 1314, at the time of the three reigns, against a man of *Gyoku-jo*. Then, coming into contact with the Chinese martial art techniques, the *kama-jutsu* evolved to the present. The technique consists of using two scythes together. A variant of the *kama-jutsu* uses two scythes linking them to the wrists with a little cord (*himo-tuki- nichōgama*); sometimes it is possible to hide a *kama* in the belt on the back. The *kama* technique is so efficient that even the sword experts tried to avoid to fight with an expert of this weapon.

The blade and the handle of the *kama* make a 90° angle. Using two *kama* (*nichō-gama*) together, it is possible to create, with the blades, angles suitable for every need, creating a scissor effect to attack and cut various parts of the body.

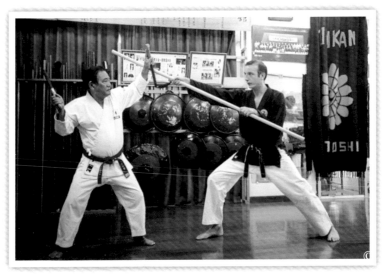

*Kōdōkan Dōjō: Shinpō Matayoshi Sensei (kama) and the author (bō)*

The most common techniques consist of hooking, cutting, and hitting using every part of the *kama*. Occasionally it could be thrown against an enemy.

The *kama* techniques come from *Chokuho Agena* taught to *Shinkō Matayoshi*, and it became his favorite weapon. For his great mastery he has been dubbed "*Kama nu ti Mateshi*" (*Matayoshi* hand of scythe).

## SCHOOL PROGRAM

The classical *kata* of the school have been simply called *Kama nu ti* (scythe techniques), there are many variants of this *kata*, but the standardized form of

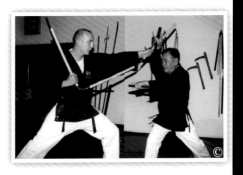

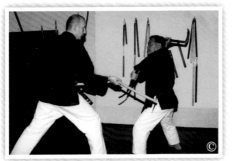

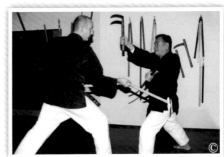

又吉古武道之武器

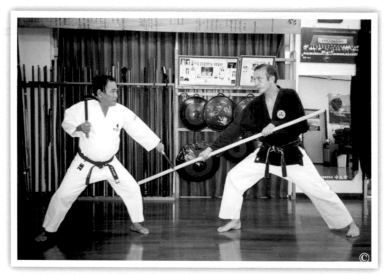

*Kōdōkan Dōjō: Shinpō Matayoshi Sensei (kama) and the author (bō)*

又吉古武道之武器

master *Matayoshi* has been repeatedly showed by *Yoshiaki Gakiya*, whom the master defined as "the best *kama* practitioner of Okinawa."

A form of *himo-tuki nichogama* was used in the period between the 1960s and the 1970s most of all for demonstrative reasons or as a traditional dance exercise.

author has creat-*hojoundō* of five techniques, as well as a base *kata* called *Kama kihon kata*.

## 鉄甲術 TEKKO

Originally the *tekko*, which means iron hand or iron metacarpus, was a horse stirrup, which was readily available and easy to transform into a very efficient knuckleduster (brass knuckle). The *tekko* was also a weapon that could be easily hidden or transported.

The *tekko* was popular as a streetfighting weapon since the 1920s, but it became officially a weapon for the *Okinawan Kobudō* only in 1934, when *Shinkō Matayoshi* brought some models of this weapon from China. He adapted to this tool some techniques of the local *Ti*; these techniques became the basis of the *tekko* of the *Matayoshi* School.

The use in pairs of the *tekko* share similiarities with some Chinese traditional weapons such as the "cogged sabers moon-sun" (*R Yue Ya Dao*), the "moon cogged ferrules" (*Yue Ya Ci*) and the "combs of the sky pal-

**Okinawan Kobudō**　　　　　　　　*History and Techniques*

ace" (*Gong Tian Shu*).

## SCHOOL PROGRAM

The handling of this weapon has been shown by master Matayoshi to very few students. No *kata* of this weapon remains known today. To make up for this, some *Kobudō* masters of the nineteenth and twentieth century have created new *kata* of *tekko*, based often on the classical *Karatedō kata*. Master Matayoshi advised me to practice with the *tek-   k  o* the *Gōjū-ryū* kata *Sēsan*; he considered it    st suitable form for this weapon.

tos published in this book that show master Shinpō Matayoshi executing *tekko* techniques are one of a kind.

## 鉄柱術 TECCHU

Most models of *tecchu* in Okinawa were imported from China. Usually this weapon is made of iron, but there are also some wooden models. Its origin is unknown, although there is a Chinese *tecchu* model which comes from a tool, which was used by the fishermen to repair the nets. Another Chinese model come from the *Emei* zone and it is called *Emei-ci* o r    *Emei-zhen* (*Emei* ferrule).

This weapon was initially known for fighting in water and it was used in pairs.

Moreover in Micronesia there is a similar weapon called a "shark knuckle," made of mangrove wood, on which shark teeth are set.

It is an unusual weapon, but easily concealable and often used as a

91

又吉古武道之武器

 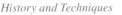

throwing weapon.

The *tecchu* has different shapes and lengths according to schools and masters who have shared the techniques and it is always used in pairs.

The *tecchu* is primarily used to make more efficient some techniques that are commonly used in *Karatedō*. For this reason the *tecchu* is considered by many people to be a complementary tool of *Karatedō* instead of a real weapon in its own right.

### SCHOOL PROGRAM

The handling of this weapon has been shown only to a few students of the school and, like the *tekko*, no classical *kata* have been retained today but only a series of exercises to practice individually or in pairs. Some *kata* have been created recently while other schools have decided to practice some *Karatedō* kata with this weapon.

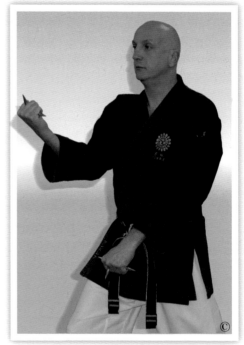

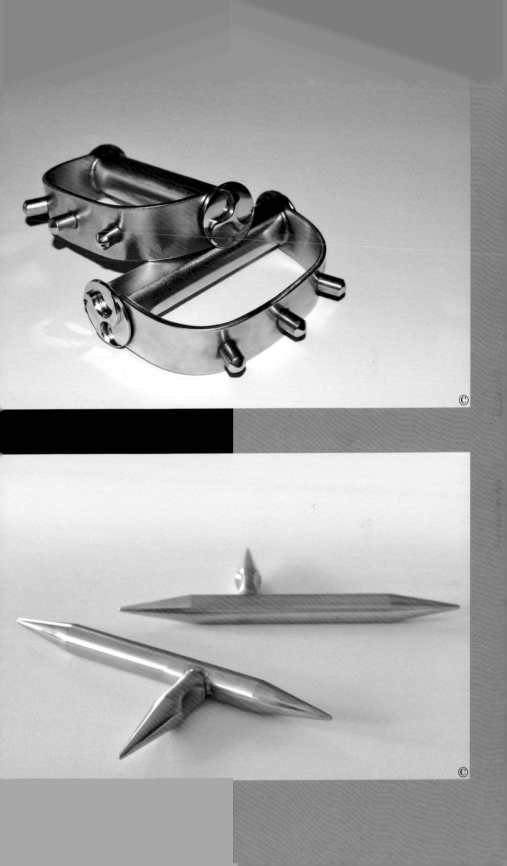

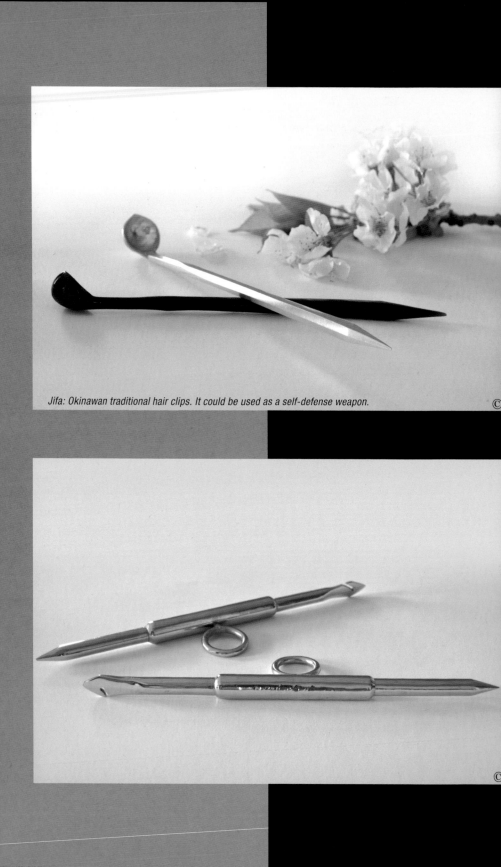

*Jifa: Okinawan traditional hair clips. It could be used as a self-defense weapon.*

# The other techniques

## INTRODUCTION

It is known that even the most advanced students of master *Shinpō Matayoshi* were not taught all the techniques that were part of the program his family acquired from many sources over the centuries.

On the occasion of the first commemorative demonstration in 1999, after the death of the master in 1997, a complete list of the known and practiced techniques was finally published. It is included here on the following pages.

This impressive list is divided in the following three groups of origin:

1. *Ryūkyū Ocho Jidai yori no Buki-jutsu*
Techniques of the weapon art of the *Ryūkyū* reign period

2. *Kingairyu Tūdi-jutsu*
Techniques of the Chinese *Kingai* School

3. *Shorinha Tsuruken* (*Go Kenki denrai*)
Techniques of the White Crane *Shaolin's* School.
(*Go Kenki's* transmission).

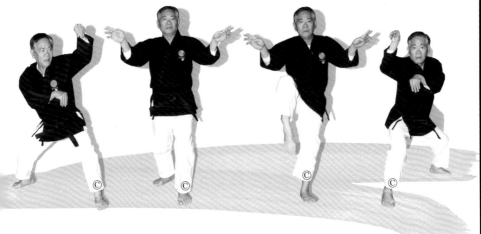

又吉古武道之武器

# FORMS OF THE WEAPON ART OF THE RYŪKYŪ REIGN EPOCH

| | WEAPON | FORMS |
|---|---|---|
| Kanji | 棒術（三尺　六尺，八尺，十二尺） | 周氏之棍，朝雲之棍，佐久川之棍，津堅之棍，漆石之棍 |
| Pronunciation | Bōjutsu(sanshaku, rokusahku, hasshaku, junishaku) | Shushi no kon, Choun no kon, Sakugawa no kon, Chikin no kon, Shiishi no kon. |
| Translation | Stick art (3 feet, 6 feet, 8 feet, 12 feet) | Shushi's stick, Choun, Sakugawa, Chikin e Shiishi Sakugawa, Chikin e Shiishi. |
| Kanji | 櫂術 （ウェーク） | 津堅赤人之櫂之手 |
| Pronunciation | Ēku-jutsu | Chikin Akachu nu Eku nu Di |
| Translation | Oar art | Oar techniques of the red man of Chikin |
| Kanji | 鍬術 | 鍬之手 |
| Pronunciation | Kuwa–jutsu | Kuwa nu ti |
| Translation | Hoe art | Hoe techniques |
| Kanji | 鎌術：一丁鎌，二丁鎌，月鎌 | 長鎌之手，鎌之手，チチ |
| Pronunciation | Kama-jutsu: Icchogama, Nichogama, Getsugama | Cho Kama nu ti, Kama nu ti, Chichi |
| Translation | Scythe art: unique double and as a moon. | Kama techniques |
| Kanji | 柱拐術 （トンクワァー） | 柱拐第一 ，柱拐第二 |
| Pronunciation | Tunkuwa–jutsu | Tunkuwadaiichi, Tunkuwa dai ni |
| Translation | Art of the rotating cylinder | Tunkuwa first, Tunkuwa second |
| Kanji | 釵術 | 二丁釵，三丁釵，千原之釵 |
| Pronunciation | Sai–jutsu | Nichosai,Sanchosai, Shinbaru no sai |
| Translation | Art of the ornamental hairpin | Double sai, triple sai, sai of the hundreds fields |
| Kanji | スルチン術 – ウニスルチン術 | No codified forms Only handling techniques |
| Pronunciation | Suruchin-jutsu | |
| Translation | Cordwith stone | |
| Kanji | 双節棍 （ヌンチャク之） | 双節棍之型 |
| Pronunciation | Sōsetsukon no kata | Sōsetsukon no kata |
| Translation | Two sections stick | Form of the two sections stick |

©

| | WEAPON | FORMS |
|---|---|---|
| Kanji | 三節棍：（大，中，小） | 三節棍之型 |
| Pronunciation | Sansetsukon (Dai, Chu, Sho) | Sansetsukon no kata |
| Translation | Three sections stick (big, medium, small) | Form of the three sections stick |
| Kanji | 四節棍 | No codified forms |
| Pronuncia | Yonsetsukon | Only handling techniques |
| Translation | Stick of four sections | |
| Kanji | 車棒 | 車棒之型 |
| Pronunciation | Kurumanbō | Kurumanb no kata |
| Translation | Rotating stick | Form of the rotating stick |
| Kanji | 籐牌 (ティンベー) | 籐牌之型 |
| Pronunciation | Tinbē | Tinbē no kata |
| Translation | Cane shield | Form with the cane shield |
| Kanji | 鉄甲術 | No codified forms |
| Pronunciation | Tekko–jutsu | Only handling techniques |
| Translation | Art of the iron nails | |
| Kanji | 鉄杜術 | No codified forms |
| Pronunciation | Tecchu–jutsu | Only handling techniques |
| Translation | Art of the iron cylinder | |

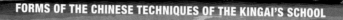

# 金代流唐手術ノ型
## KINGAIRYŪ TŌDE-JUTSU ＝ KATA

### FORMS OF THE CHINESE TECHNIQUES OF THE KINGAI'S SCHOOL

©

| KANJI | PRONUNCIATION | TRANSLATION |
|---|---|---|
| 三戦 | Sanchin | 3 conflicts |
| 王冠 | Okan (Wankan) | King crown |
| 十三 | Sesan | 13 |
| 五十四 | Gojushi (Useshi) | 54 |
| 五十七 | Gojunana | 57 |
| 虎法 | Koho (Tora ho) | Tiger method |
| 虎鶴 | Kotsuru (Tora tsuru) | Tiger and crane |
| 貫手術 | Nunti-jutsu | Art of the piercing techniques (lance) |
| 藤牌 | Tinbei (Tohai) | Shield |
| 流 | Ryuchin (Suruchin) | Cord with loads |
| 手裏剣術 | Shuriken-jutsu | Art of the throwing weapons |

N.B.: *The reported terminology has been written by M° Matayoshi, without any variation, where, sometimes, the term "jutsu" has been omitted.*

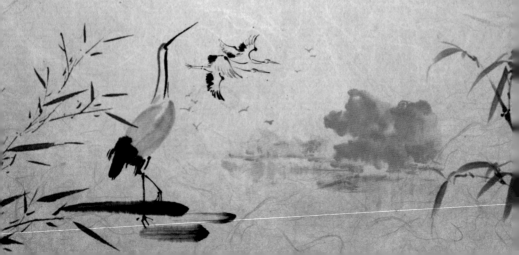

# 少林派鶴拳（呉賢貴伝系）－型
## SHORINHA TSURUKEN (GO KENKI DENRAI) – KATA

**FORMS OF THE WHITE CRANE SCHOOL OF SHAOLIN (GO KENKI'S TRANSMISSION)**

| KANJI | PRONUNCIATION | TRANSLATION |
|---|---|---|
| 八步連 | Papuren | 8 consecutive steps |
| 二十八 | Nepai | 28 |
| 鶴法 | Tsuruho | Crane method |
| 白鶴兵法初段之事 | Hakutsuru heiho shodan no koto | Base strategy of the White Crane |
| 白鶴兵法弐段之事 | Hakutsuru heiho nidan no koto | Intermediate strategy of the White Crane |
| 白鶴兵法参段之事 | Hakutsuru heiho sandan no koto | Advanced strategy of the White Crane |
| 白鶴双刀 | Hakutsuru soto | Double swords of the White Crane |

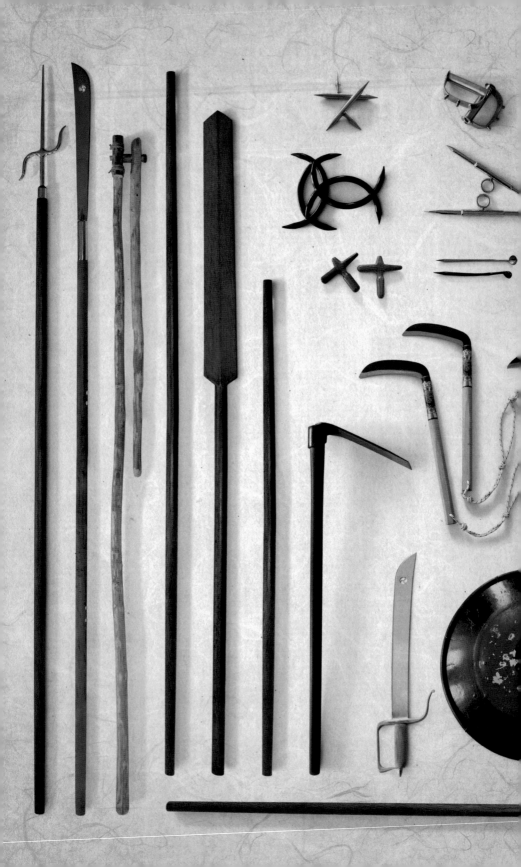

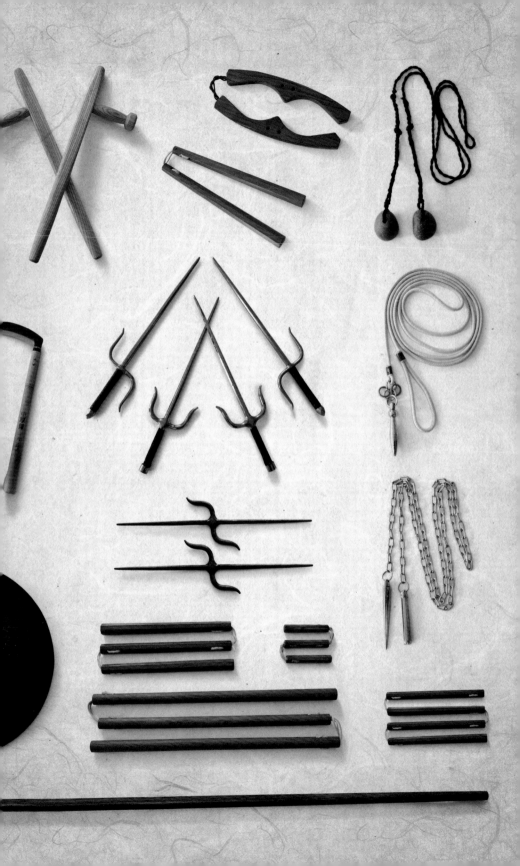

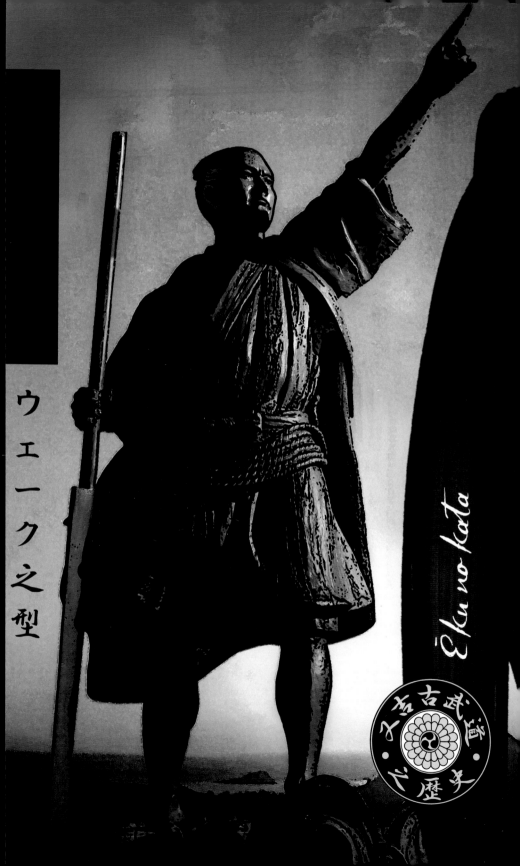

ウエーク之型

*Eku no kata*

# Introduction

*Chikin Akachu no ēkudi*, that is: techniques of the red man of *Chikin* (*jima*). The description of this weapon, its origin and the use have been discussed earlier in Chapter 2.

This *kata* was the favorite of master *Shinpō Matayoshi* and he demonstrated it on hundreds of occasions with his favorite *ēku*. The master became so fond of this weapon that the family, in accordance with his wishes, placed it near the master during the traditional cremation. The belief is that this way he can still use his beloved oar in the next world.

This *kata* encompasses all of the *ēku-jutsu* techniques of the *Matayoshi* School: *Yoko Uke*, *Osae Uke*, *Kake Uke*, *Jodan Uke*, many forms of *Zukiwaza*, *Uchi-waza*, *Tobi-waza*, *Sunakake*, and *Kamae*.

103

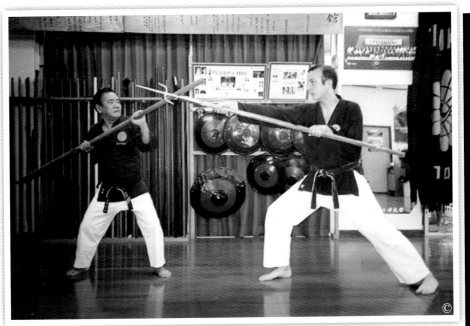

*Kōdōkan Dōjō: Shinpō Matayoshi Sensei (ēku) and the author (nunti-bō)*

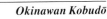

ウェーク之型

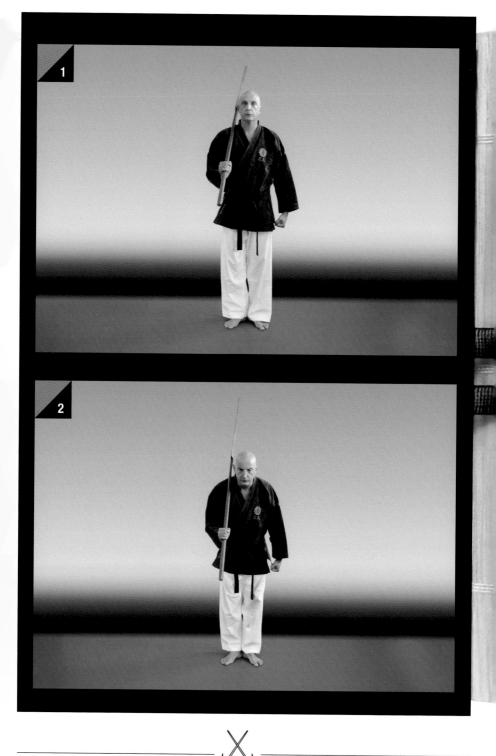

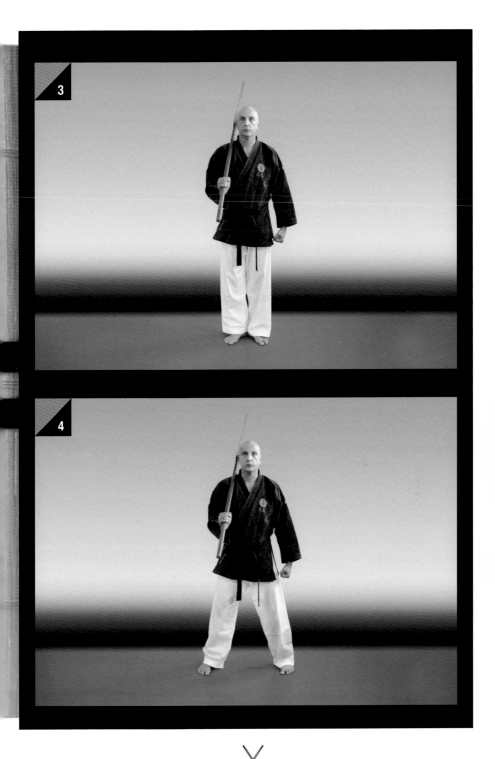

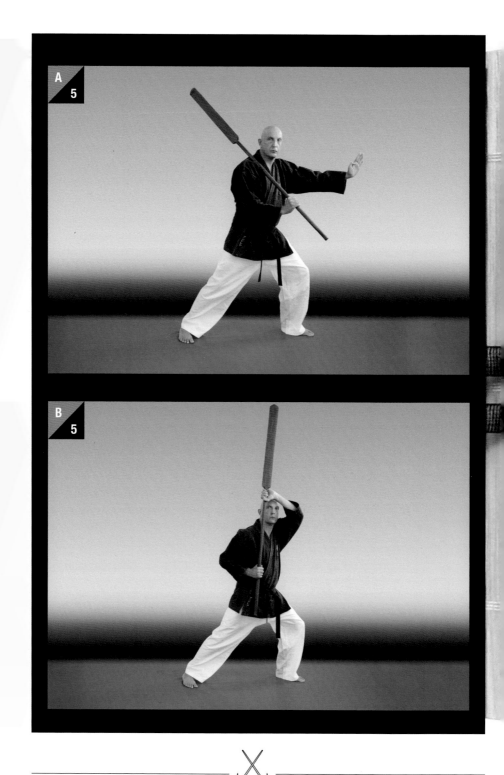

 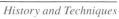

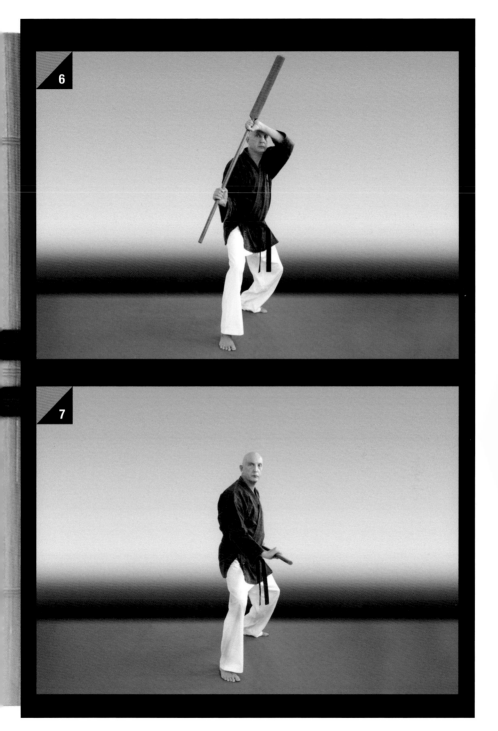

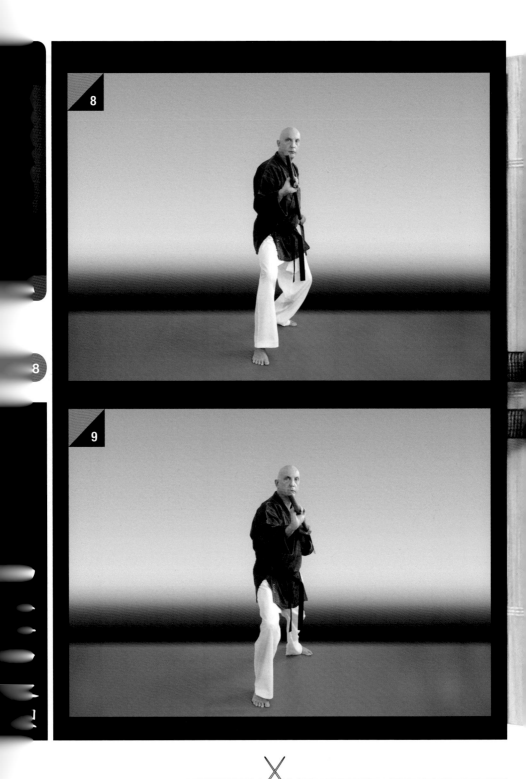

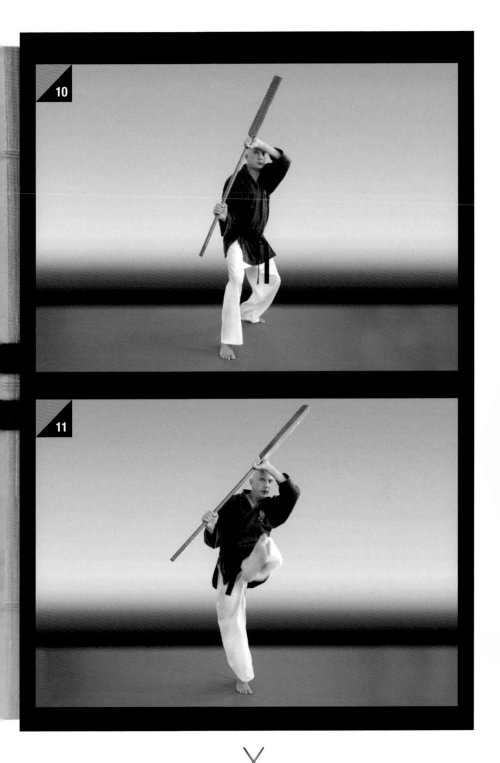

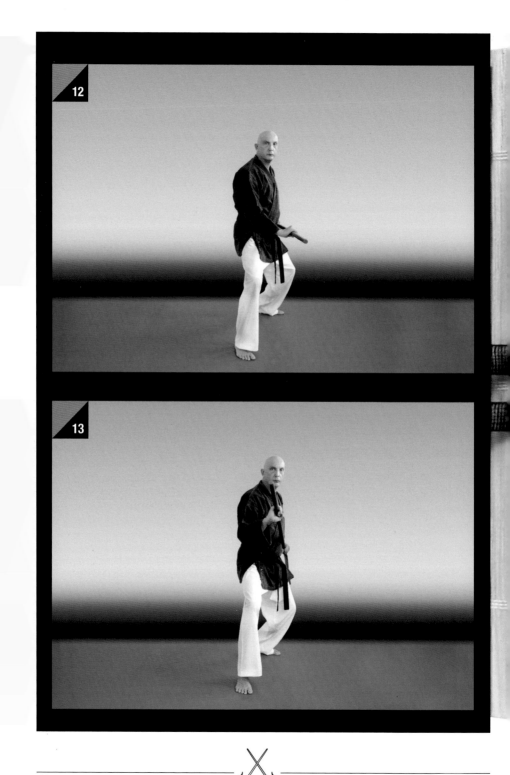

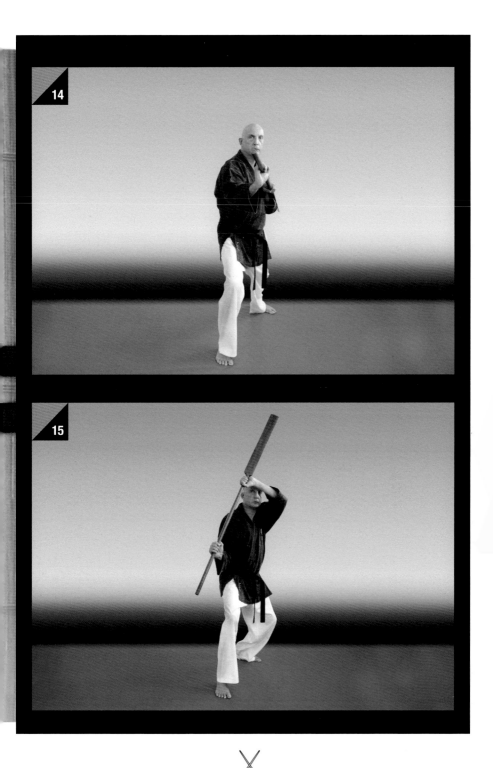

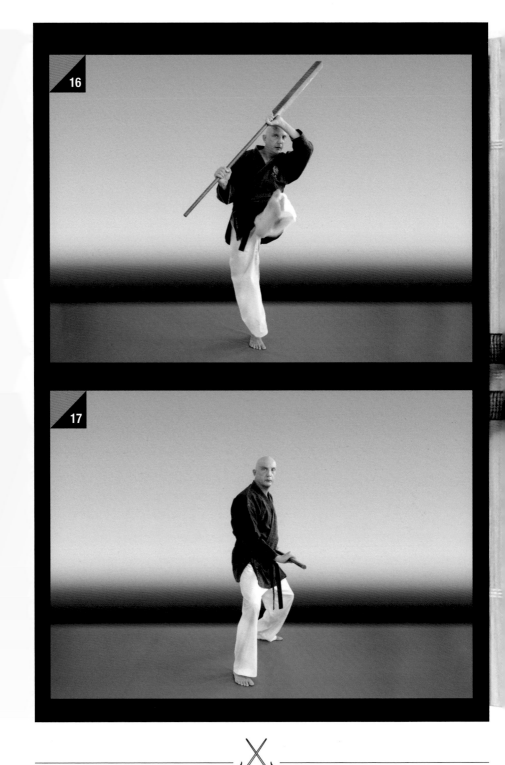

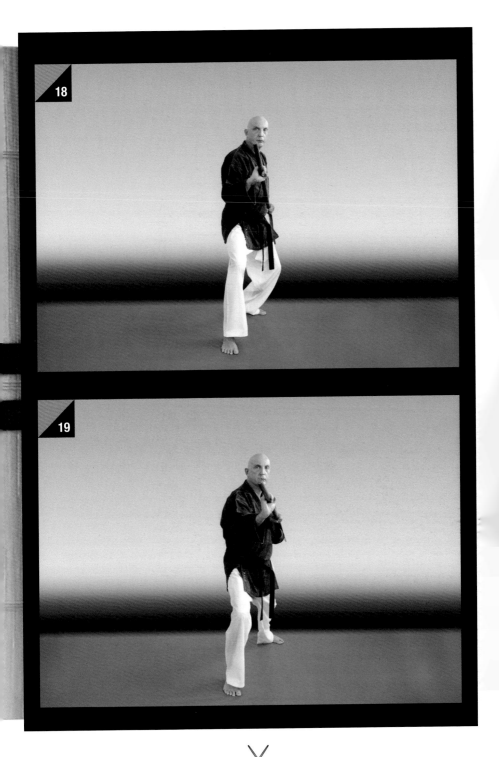

 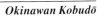

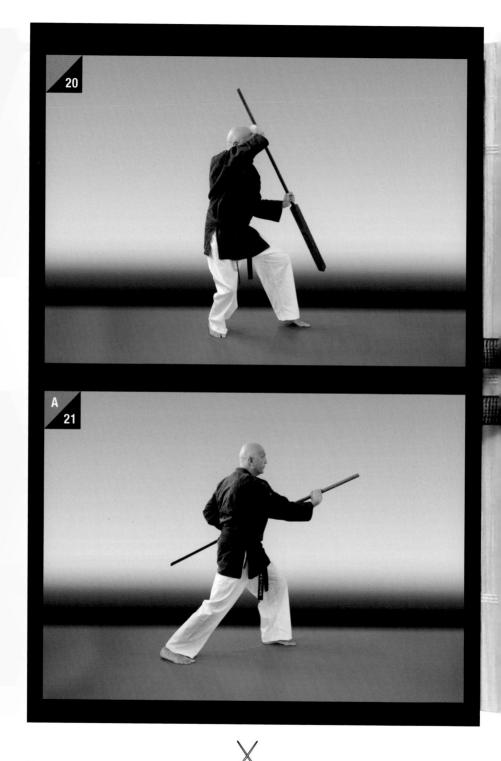

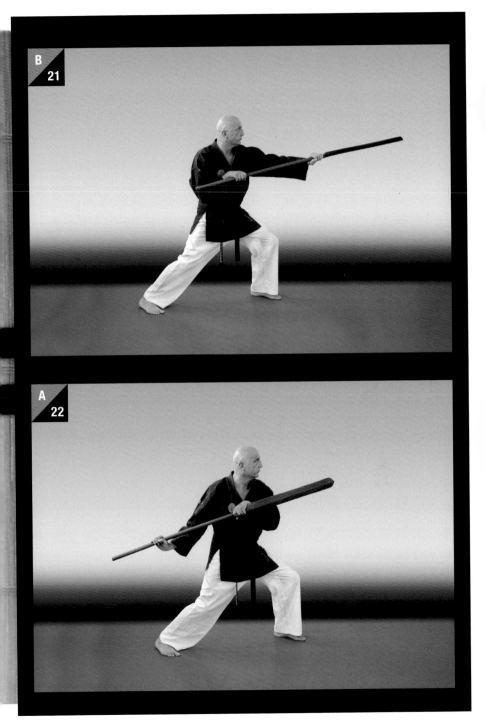

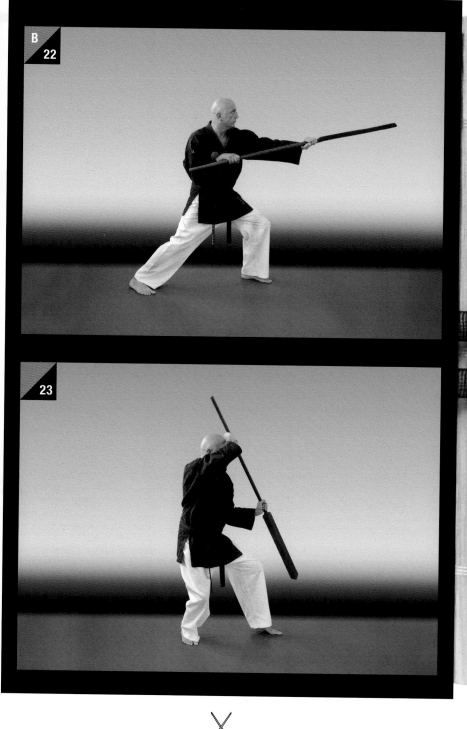

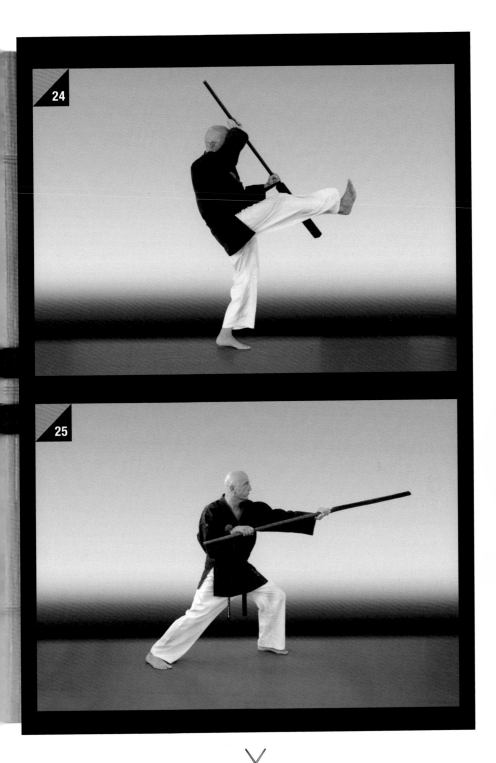

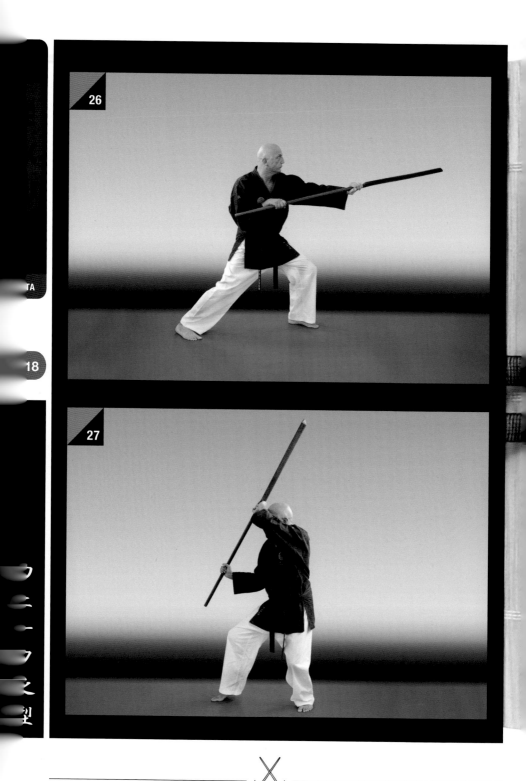

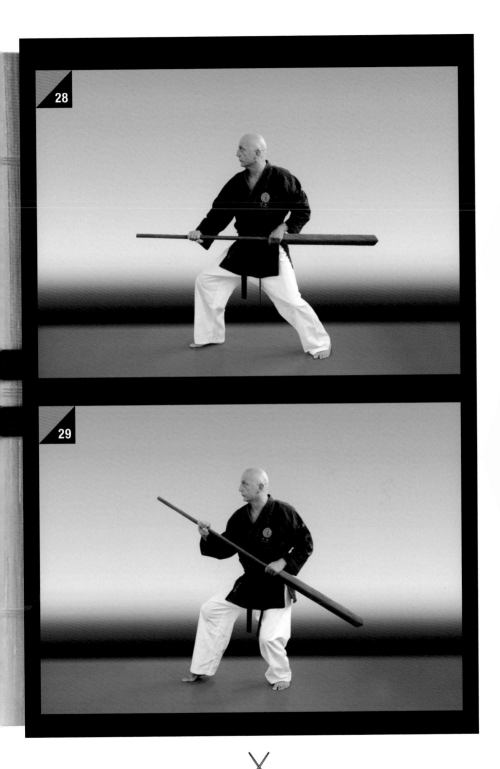

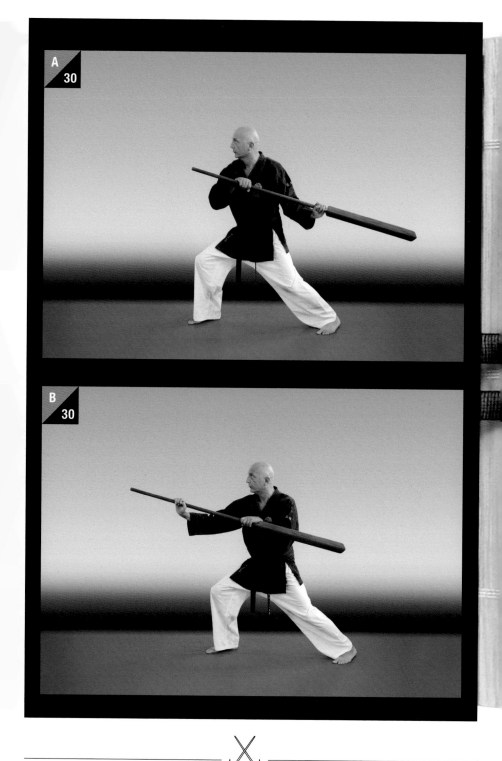

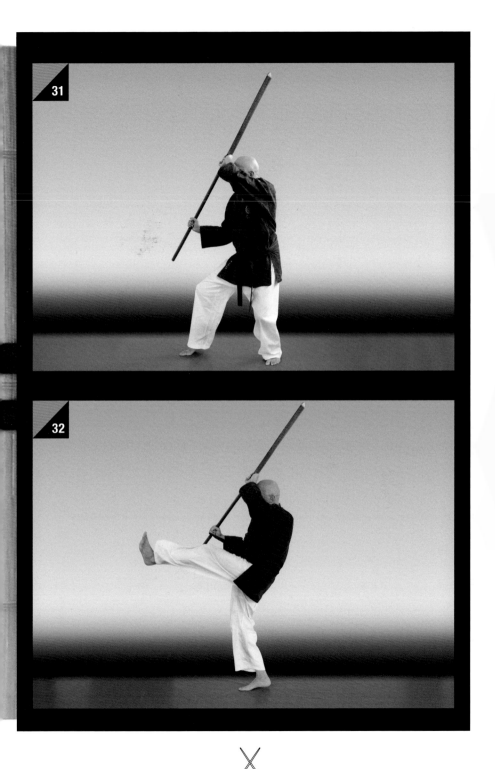

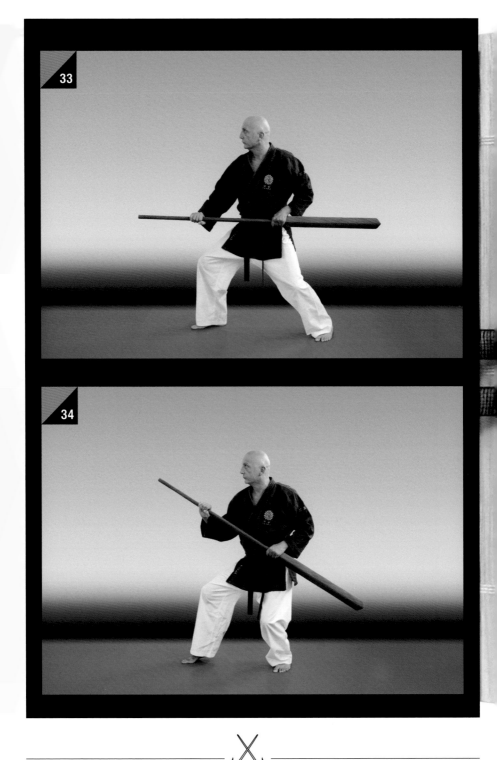

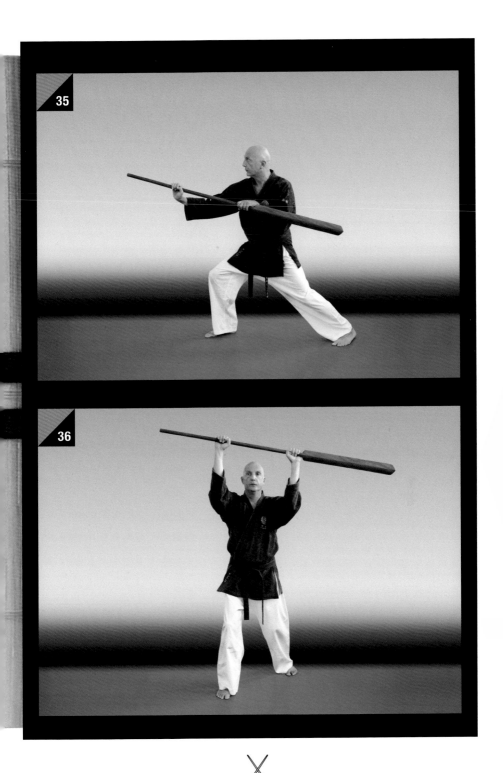

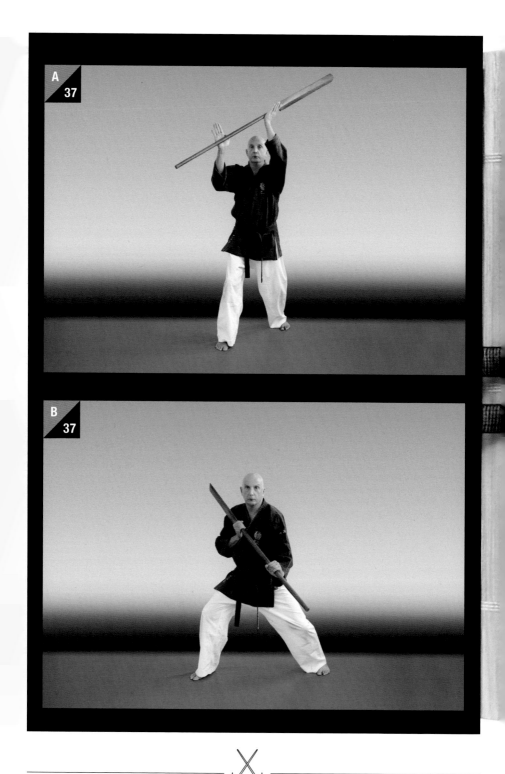

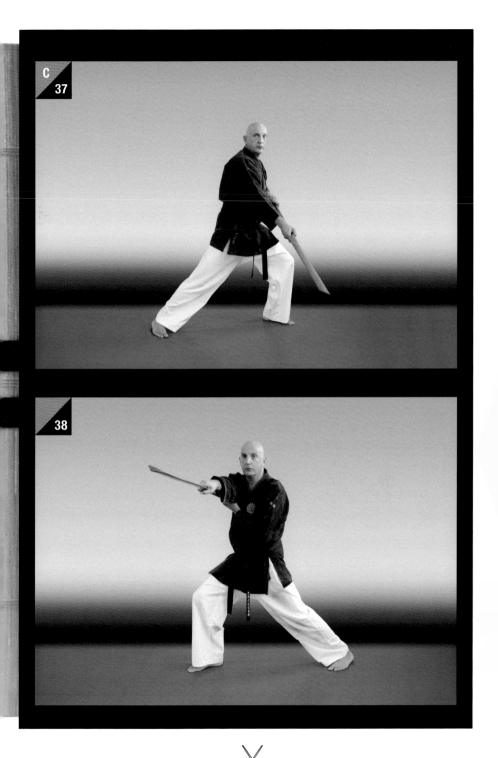

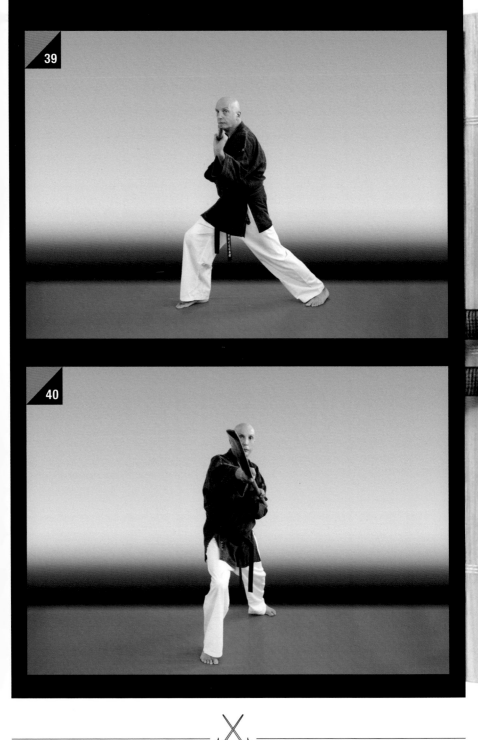

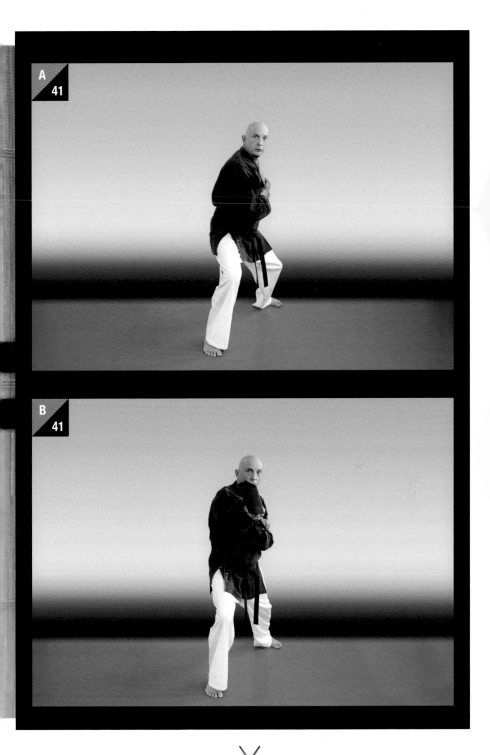

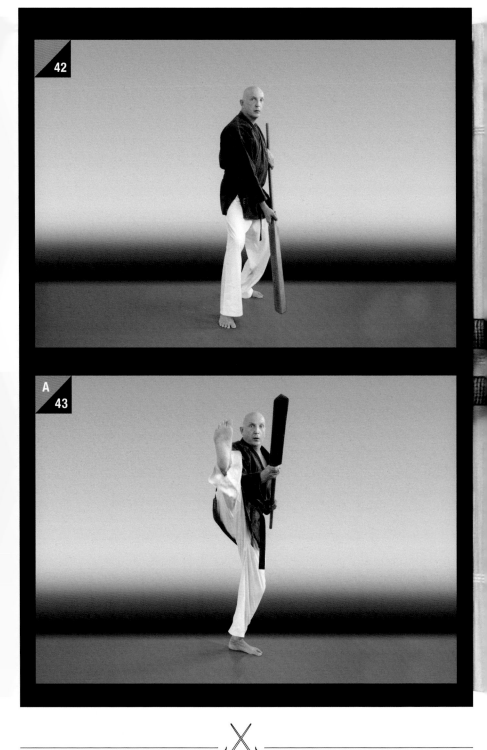

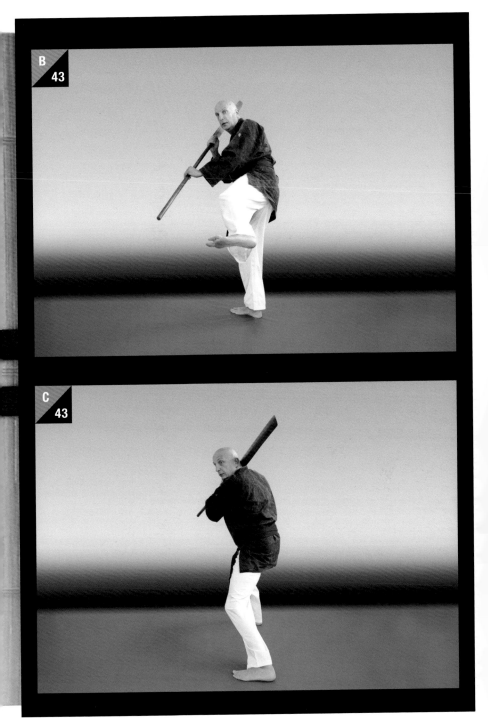

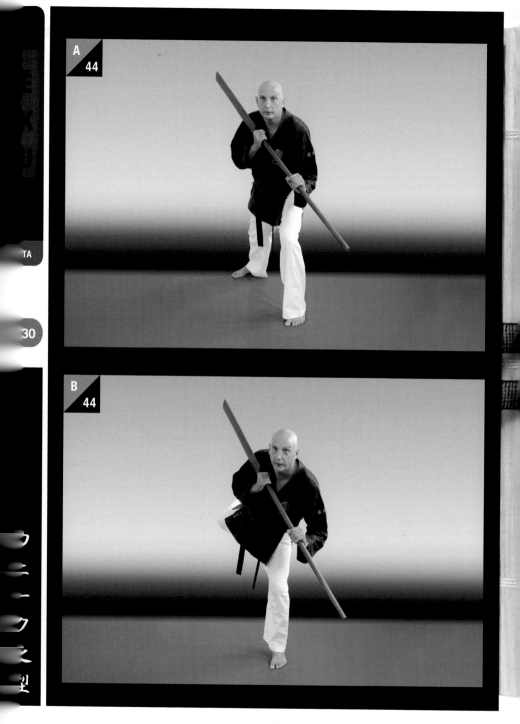

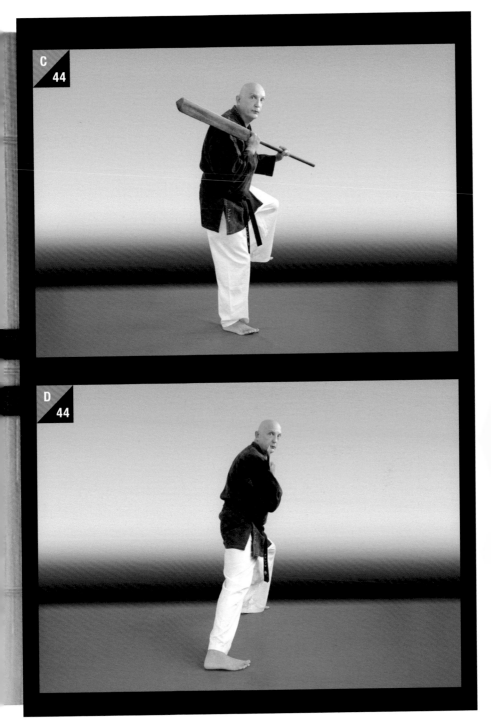

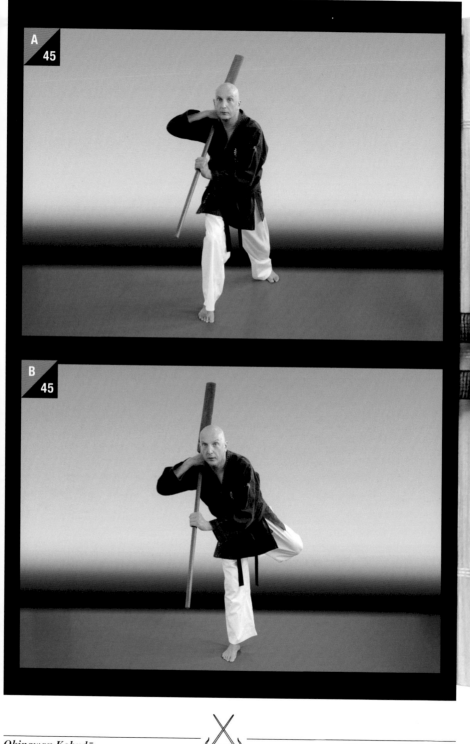

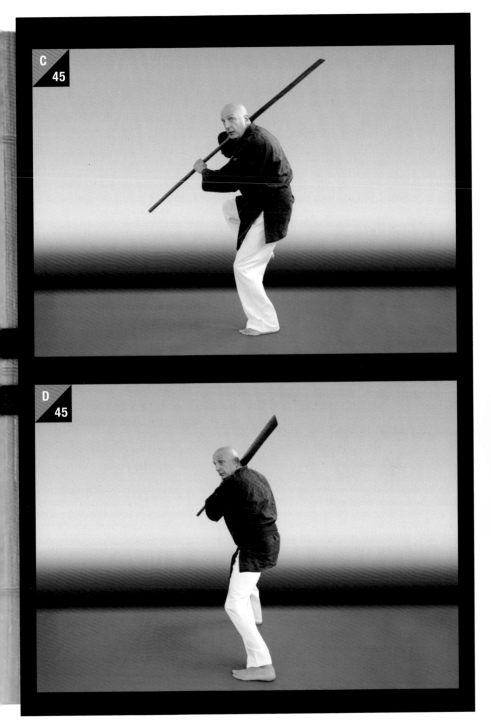

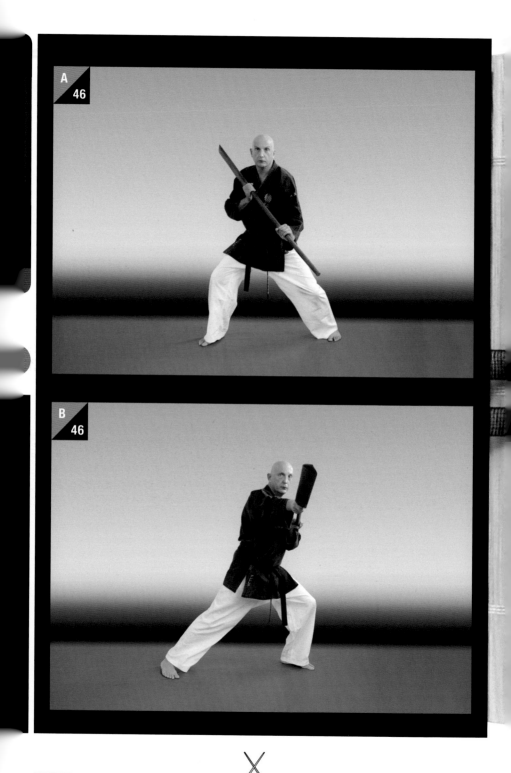

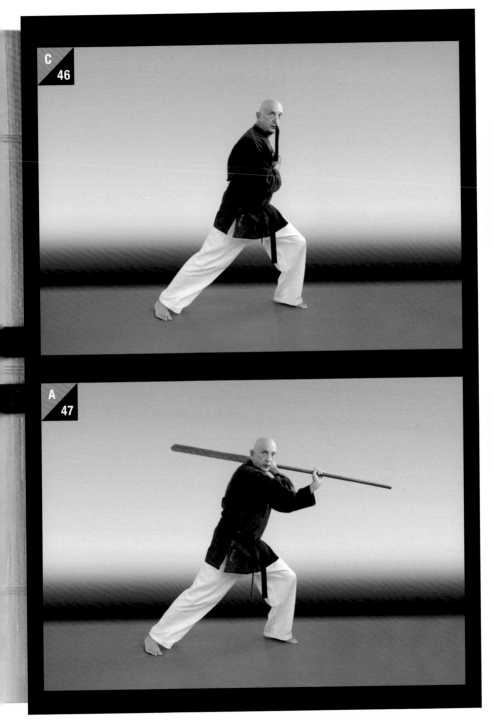

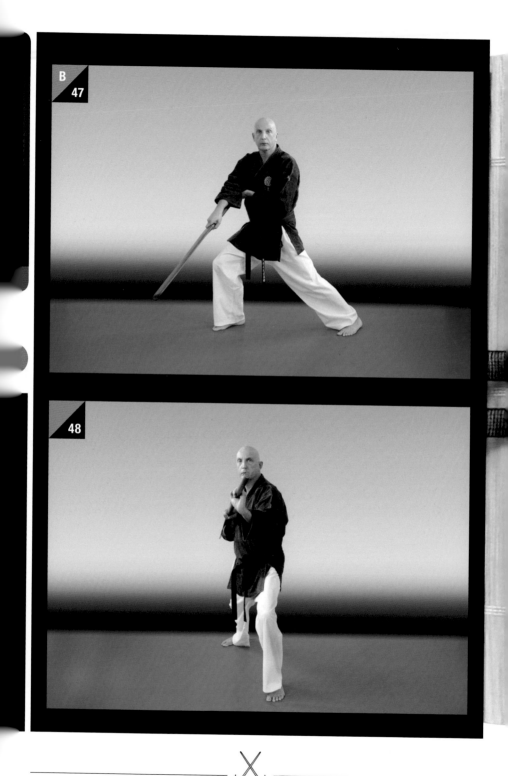

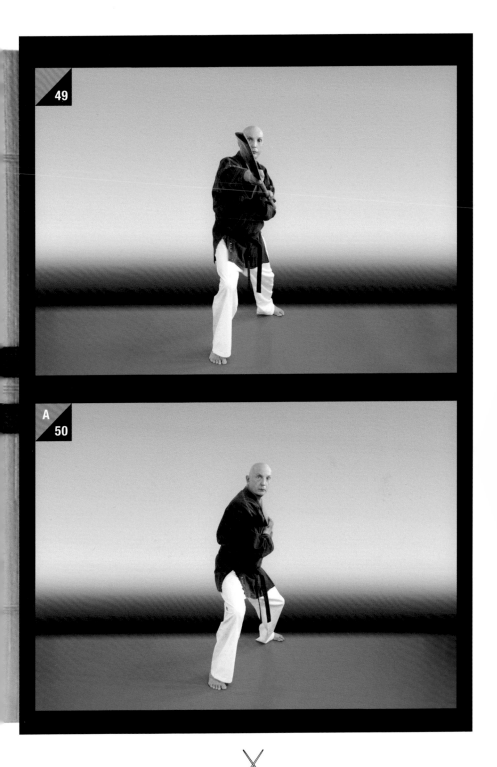

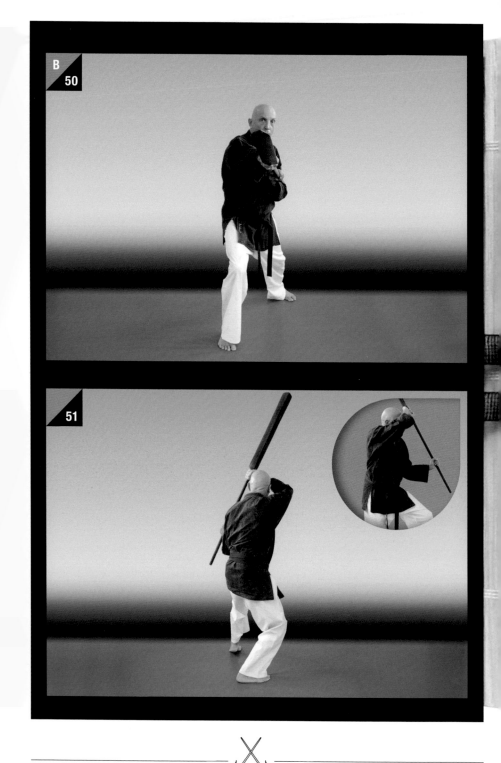

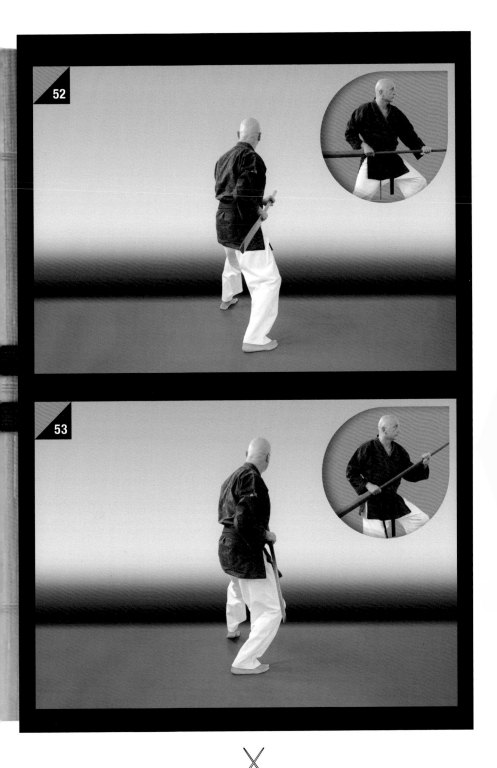

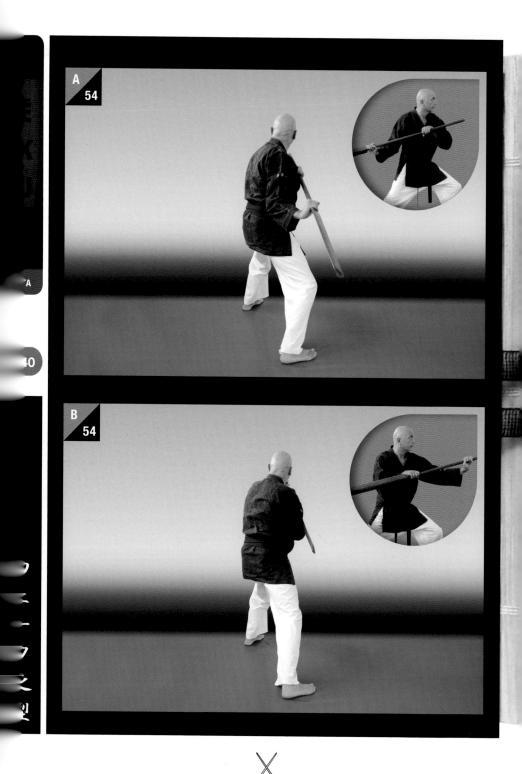

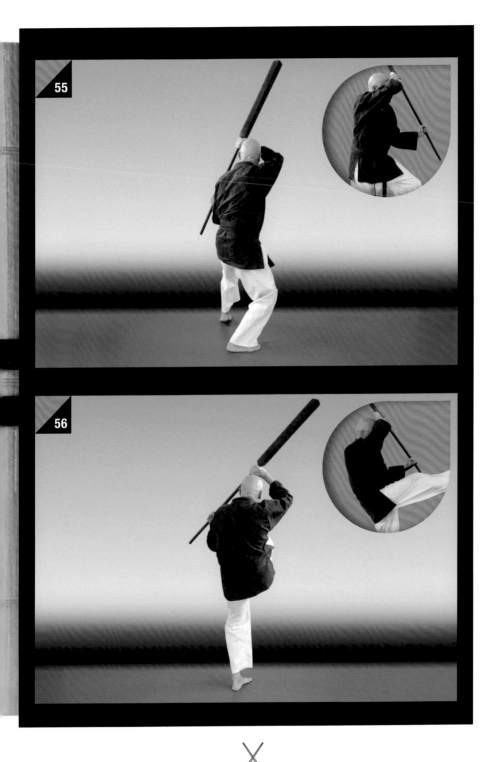

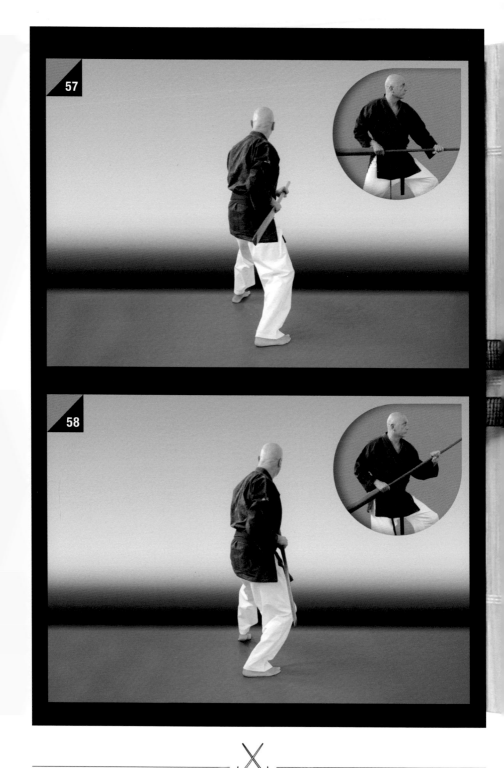

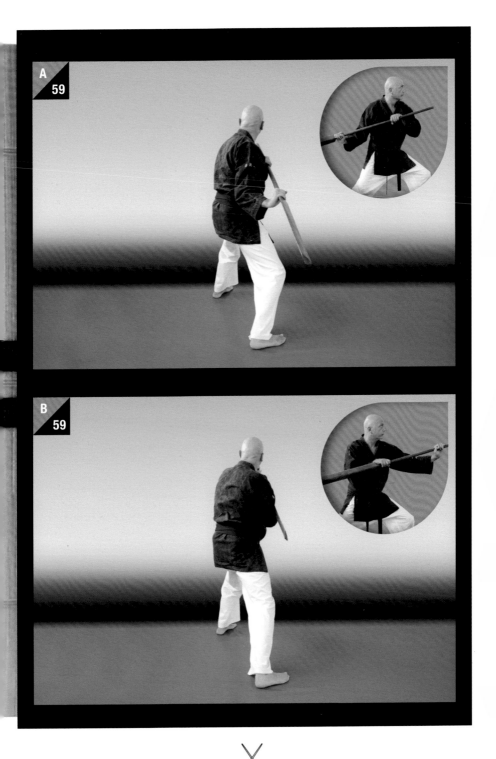

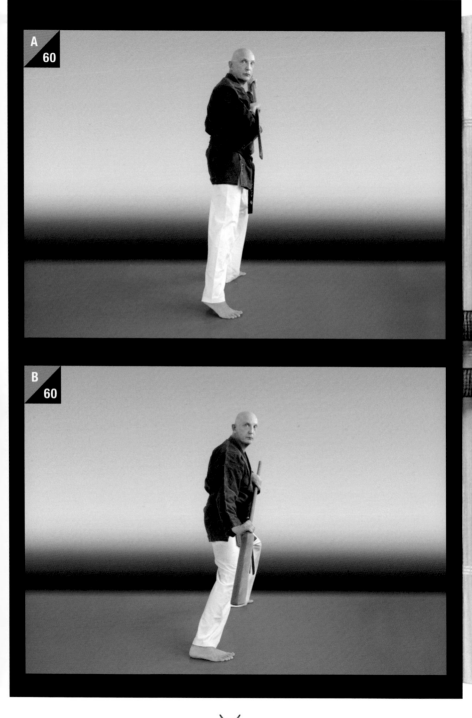

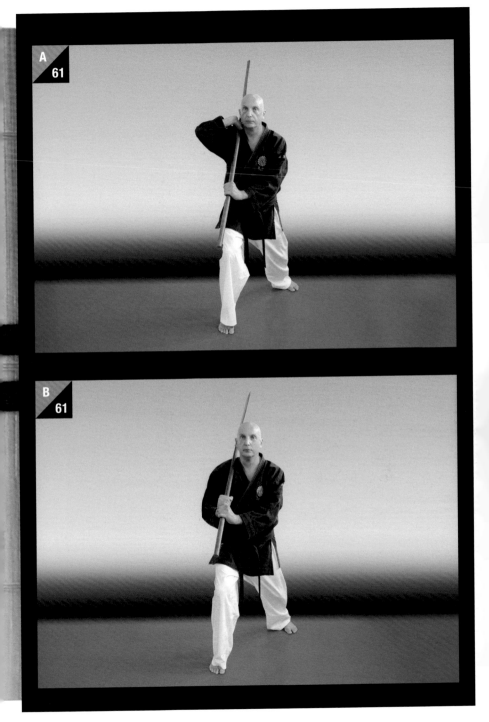

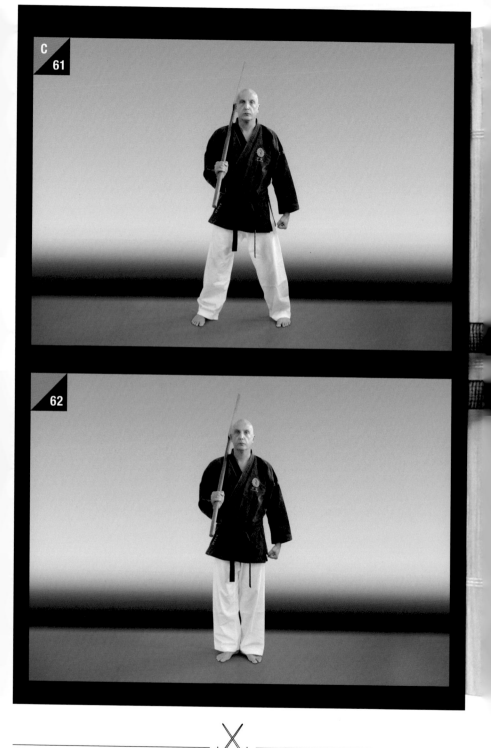

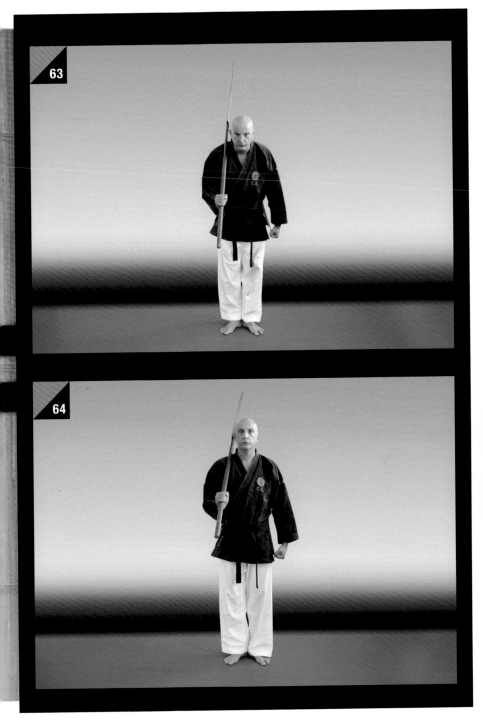

## DESCRIPTION

01. Musubi-dachi
02. Rei
03. Kiozuke
04. Move left foot: Heiko-dachi.
05. Rotate the hip. Move the Ēku to left.
    Raise the left arm and catch the oar with the left hand. Yoi no shisei.
06. Go ahead with the left foot in Hanmi neko-ashi dachi. Yoko-uke.
07. Lay the right heel. Osae-uke.
08. Withdraw the right in Hanmi neko-ashi dachi. Kake-uke.
09. Go ahead with the right in Zenkuzu dachi. Kaeshi-zuki.
10. Withdraw the right in Hanmi neko-ashi dachi. Yoko-uke.
11. Left Sunakake.
12. Lay the left in front of the right.
    Go ahead with the right. Osae-uke.
13. Repeat 8.
14. Repeat 9.
15. Repeat 10.
16. Repeat 11.
17. Repeat 12.
18. Repeat 8.
19. Repeat 9.

### Direction change
20. Go to left with the left.
    Hanmi neko-ashi dachi. Gedan yoko-uke.
21. Go ahead with the left in Zenkuzu dachi. Age naname-uchi.
22. On place, Jodan-zuki.
23. Withdraw the left in Hanmi neko-ashi dachi. Gedan yoko-uke.
24. Right Sunakake.
25. Lay the right in front of the left.
    Go ahead with the left. Age naname-uchi.
26. Repeat 22

### Direction change
27. Yori-ashi to the back. Hanmi neko-ashi dachi. Yoko-uke.
28. Lay the right heel. Osae-uke.
29. Withdraw the right in Hanmi neko-ashi dachi. Kake-uke.
30. Go ahead with the right in Zenkuzu dachi. Kaeshi-zuki.
31. Withdraw the right in Hanmi neko-ashi dachi. Yoko-uke.
32. Left Sunakake.

33. Lay the left in front of the right.
    Go ahead with the right. Osae-uke.
34. Repeat 29.
35. Repeat 30.

### Direction change
36. Move the left back. Hanzenkuzu-dachi. Jodan age-uke.
37. Line up the left to the right. Change grip. Naname zenkuzu-dachi. Gedan yoko-uchi.
38. Rotate the hip. Chudan ura-uchi.
39. On place, Kaeshi-uchi.
40. Go ahead with the right in Zenkuzu dachi. Jodan naname-uchi.
41. On place, Jodan zuki.
42. Withdraw the right foot (heel up). Preparation.
43. Tobi sunakake. KIAI. Knock down in Kokuzu-dachi: Naname kokuzu kamae.
44. Tobi gedan-uke. Knock down Kokuzu-dachi: Kokuzu kamae.
45. Tobi gedan-uke. Knock Kokuzu-dachi: Naname kokuzu kamae.
46. Line up the right to the left. Naname zenkuzu-dachi. Jodan naname-uchi, Hiki-kiri.
47. Rotate the hip. Gedan ura-uchi.
48. Go ahead with the left in Zenkuzu dachi. Jodan kaeshi-uchi.
49. Go ahead with the right in Zenkuzu dachi. Jodan naname-uchi.
50. On place, Jodan zuki.

### Direction change
(repeat symmetrically the sequence from 27 to 35)
51. Yori-ashi to the back. Hanmi neko-ashi dachi. Change grip, Yoko-uke.
52. Lay the right heel. Osae-uke.
53. Withdraw the right in Hanmi neko-ashi dachi. Kake-uke.
54. Go ahead with the right in Zenkuzu dachi. Kaeshi-zuki
55. Withdraw the right in Hanmi neko-ashi dachi. Yoko-uke.
56. Left Sunakake.
57. Lay the left in front of the right.
    Go ahead with the right. Osae-uke.
58. Repeat 53.
59. Repeat 54.

### Direction change
60. Withdraw the right and pulling the Ēku go ahead with the right. Kokuzu-dachi, Ushiro gedan-zuki. KIAI.
61. Go ahead with the left in Heiko-dachi bringing back the Ēku on the right shoulder.
62. Musubi-dachi
63,64. Rei

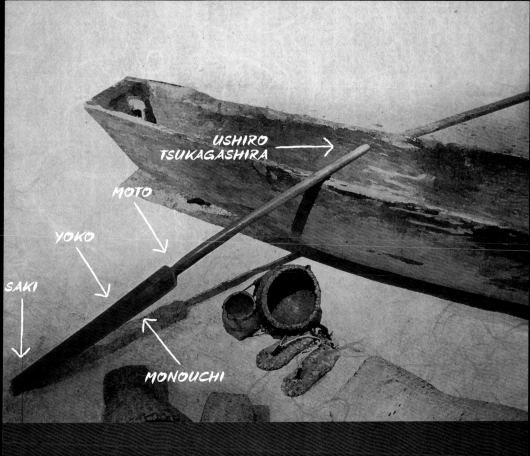

USHIRO TSUKAGASHIRA

MOTO

YOKO

SAKI

MONOUCHI

when the kata is executed during a collective lesson under the guide of a teacher, more techniques have to be executed to every one of his orders in order to connect them together. The concatenation *(renraku)* represents the rhythm of the kata which have to be respected also during the individual execution. The concatenation of *Chikin Akachu no Ekudi* is the following:

**1** - 2, 3 - **4**, 5 - 6 - 7, 8, 9, 10 - 11, 12, 13, 14, 15 - 16, 17, 18, 19, 20 - 21, 22, 23 - 24, 25, 26, 27 - 28, 29, 30, 31 - 32, 33, 34, 35, 36 - 37, 38, 39 - 40, 41, 42 - 43 - 44 - 45 - 46, 47, 48 - 49, 50, 51 - 52, 53, 54, 55 - 56, 57, 58, 59, 60 - 61 - 62 - 63, 64.

The comma divides the movements to execute with the same order, the hyphen indicates the separation between one order and another. In bold are the techniques accompanied with the **KIAI** emission.

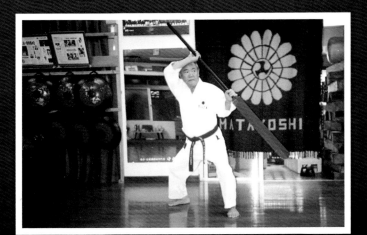

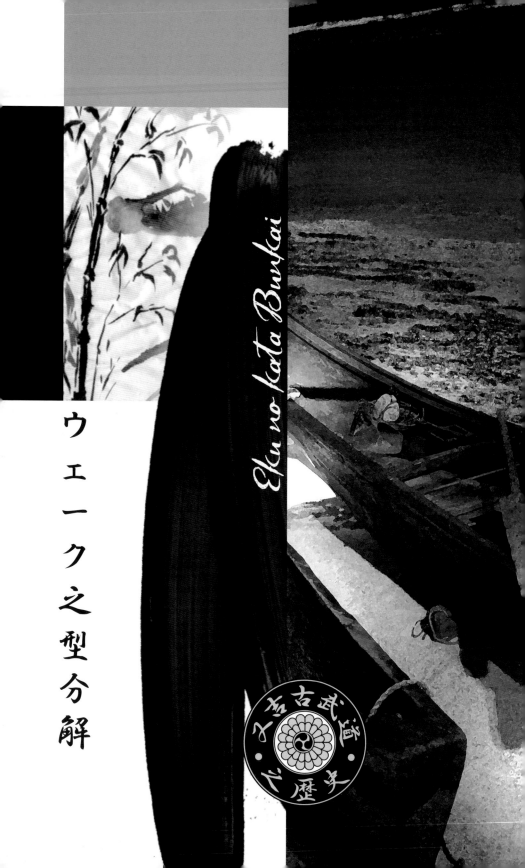

ウェイク之型分解

Eku no Kata Bunkai

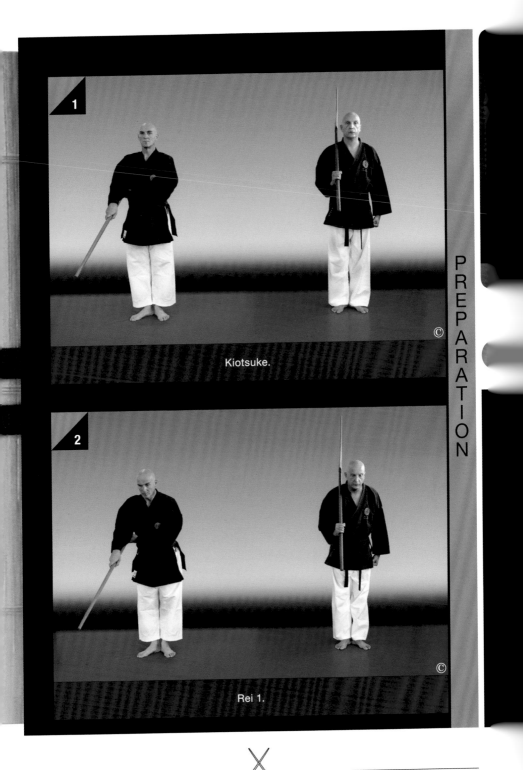

1

Kiotsuke.

2

Rei 1.

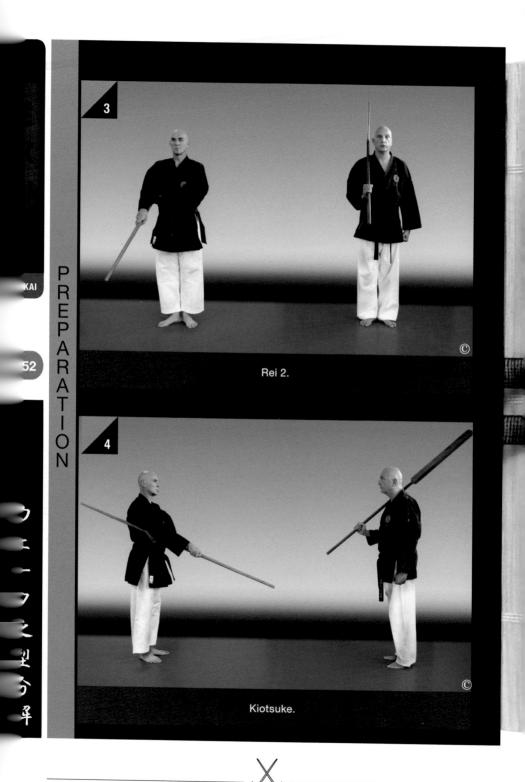

Rei 2.

Kiotsuke.

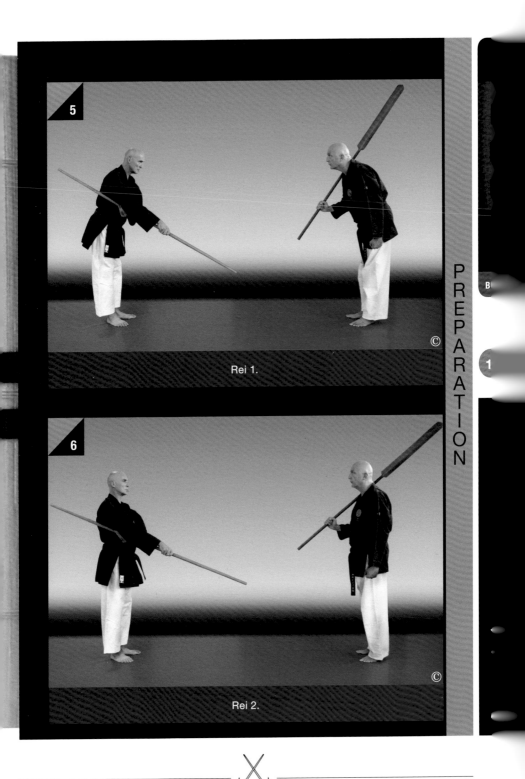

Rei 1.

Rei 2.

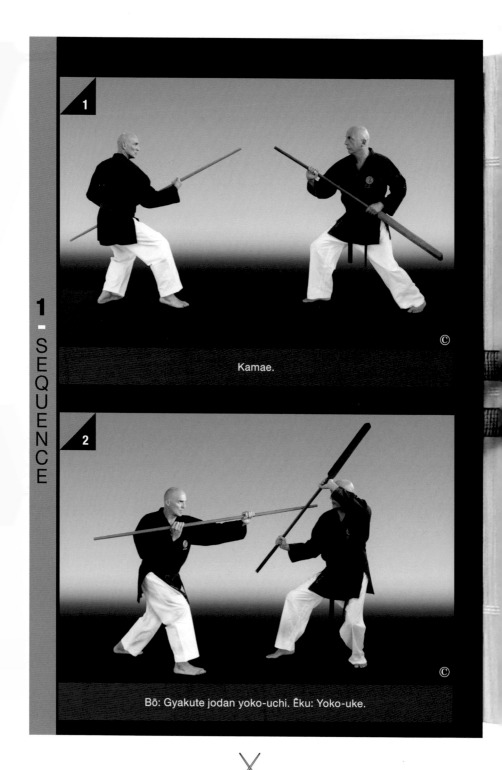

Kamae.

Bō: Gyakute jodan yoko-uchi. Ēku: Yoko-uke.

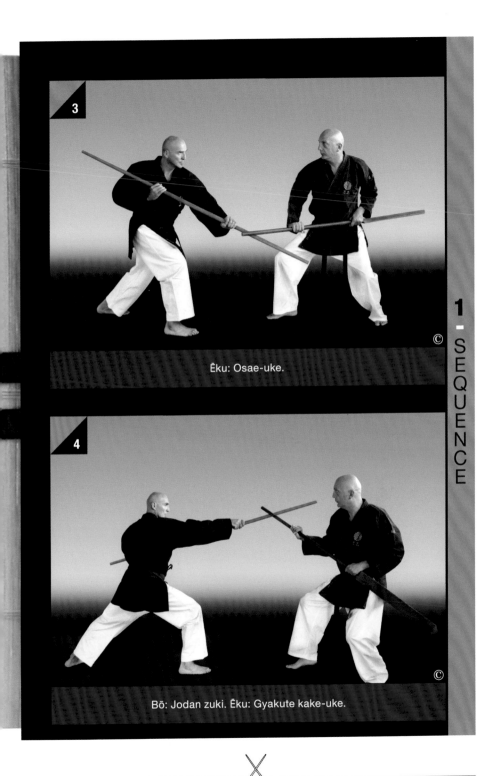

Ēku: Osae-uke.

Bō: Jodan zuki. Ēku: Gyakute kake-uke.

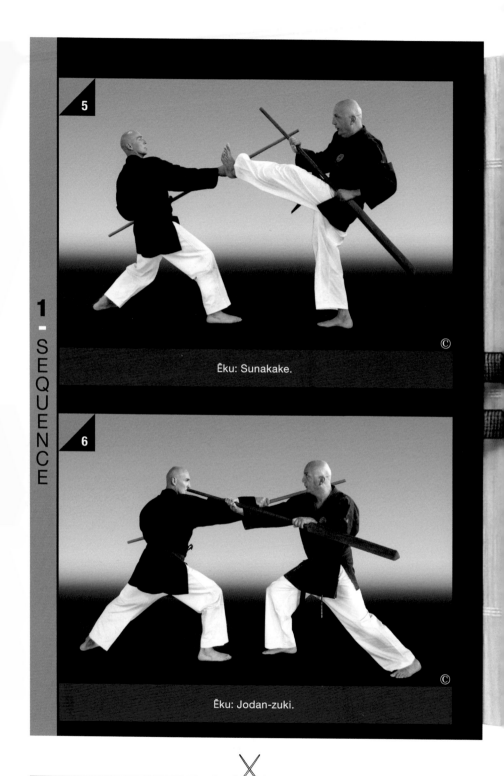

**5**

Êku: Sunakake.

**6**

Êku: Jodan-zuki.

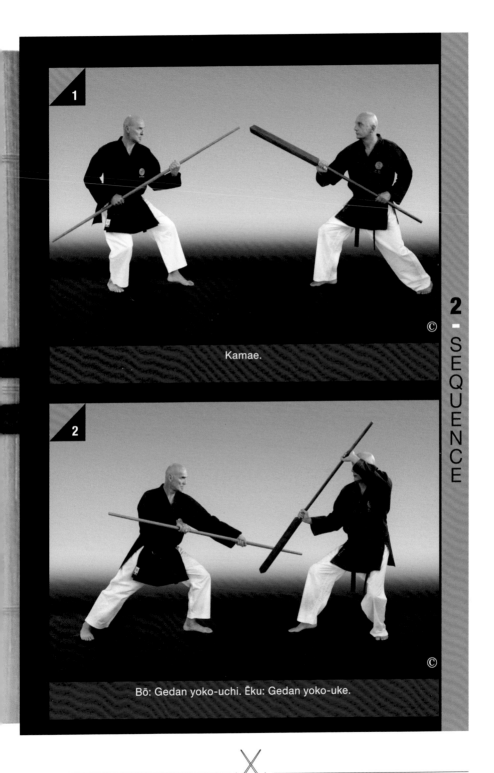

Kamae.

Bō: Gedan yoko-uchi. Ēku: Gedan yoko-uke.

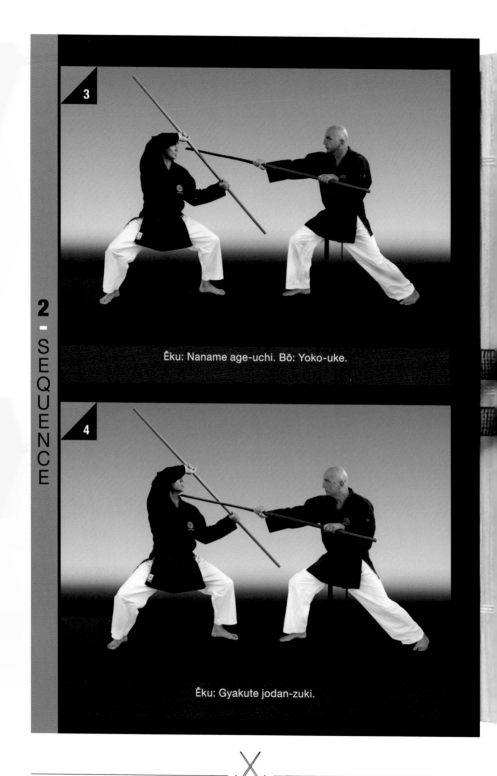

Ēku: Naname age-uchi. Bō: Yoko-uke.

Ēku: Gyakute jodan-zuki.

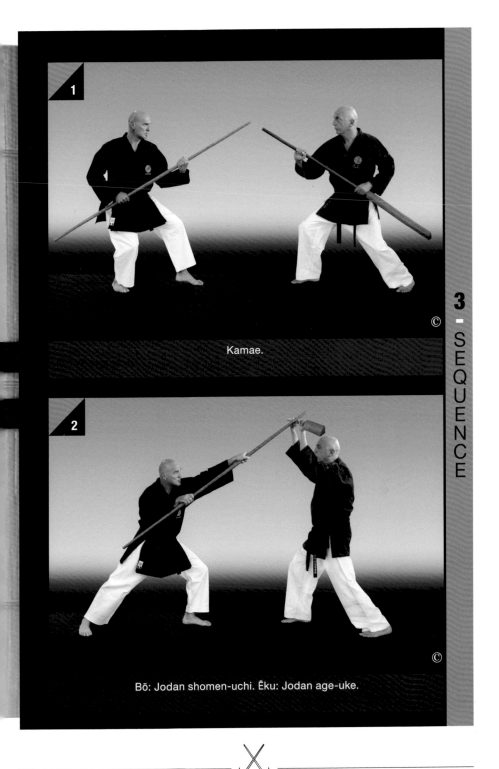

**1**

Kamae.

**2**

Bō: Jodan shomen-uchi. Ēku: Jodan age-uke.

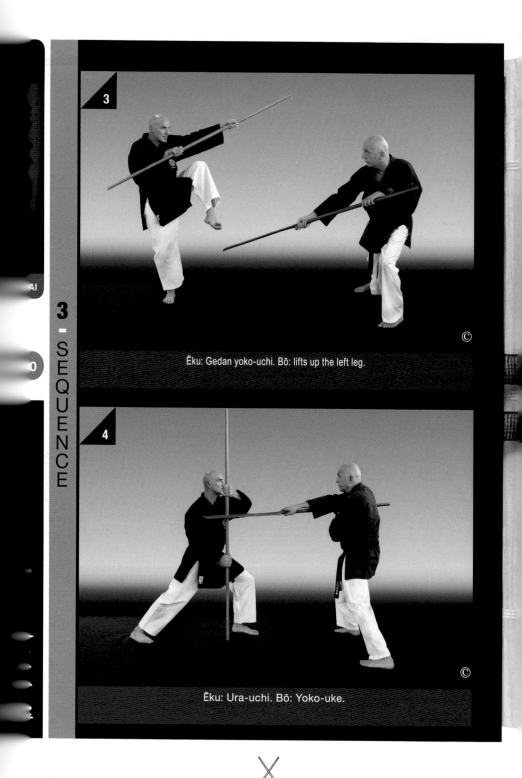

Ēku: Gedan yoko-uchi. Bō: lifts up the left leg.

Ēku: Ura-uchi. Bō: Yoko-uke.

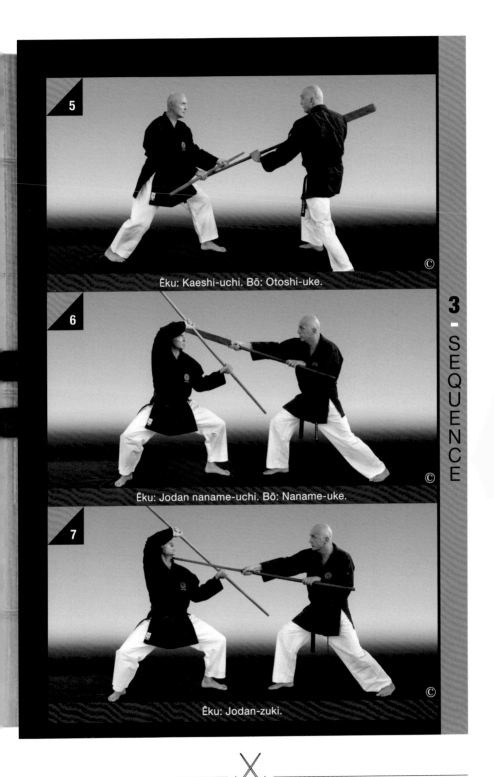

**5** Ēku: Kaeshi-uchi. Bō: Otoshi-uke.

**6** Ēku: Jodan naname-uchi. Bō: Naname-uke.

**7** Ēku: Jodan-zuki.

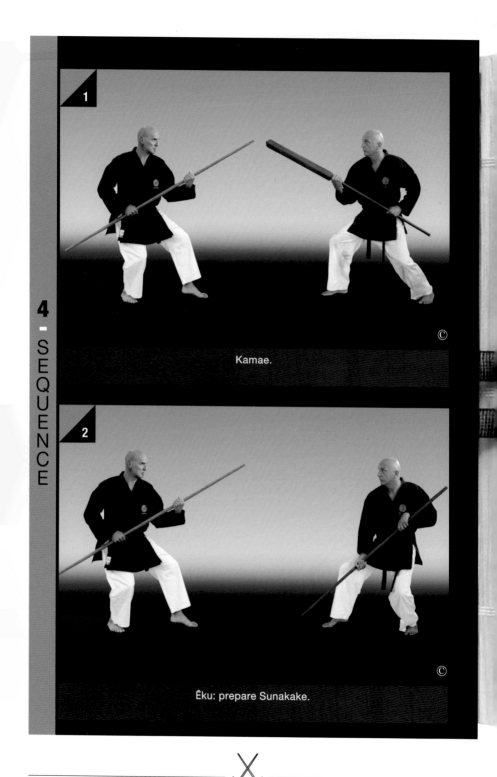

Kamae.

Êku: prepare Sunakake.

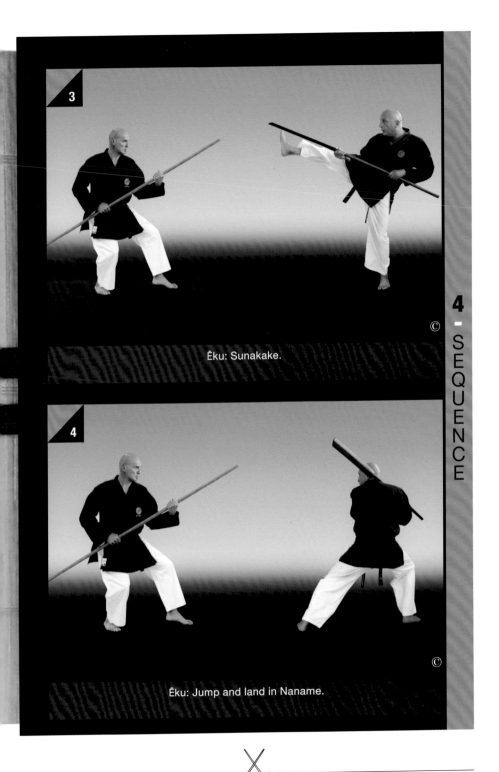

Ēku: Sunakake.

Ēku: Jump and land in Naname.

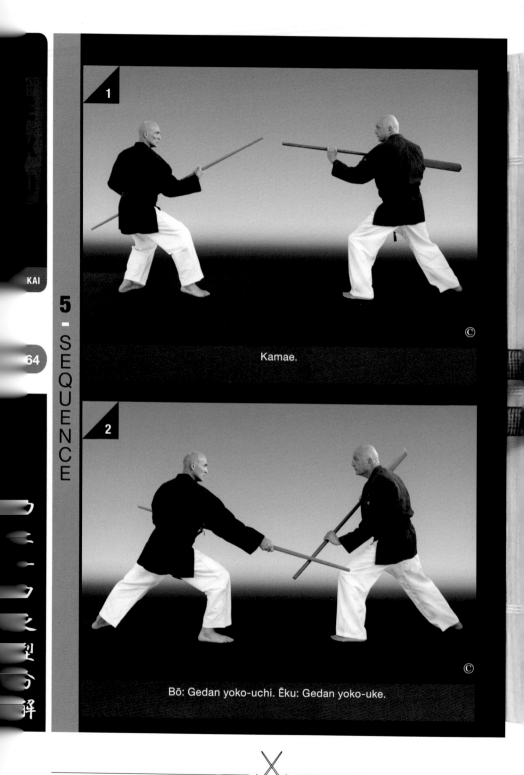

1

Kamae.

©

2

Bō: Gedan yoko-uchi. Êku: Gedan yoko-uke.

©

Okinawan Kobudō

*History and Techniques*

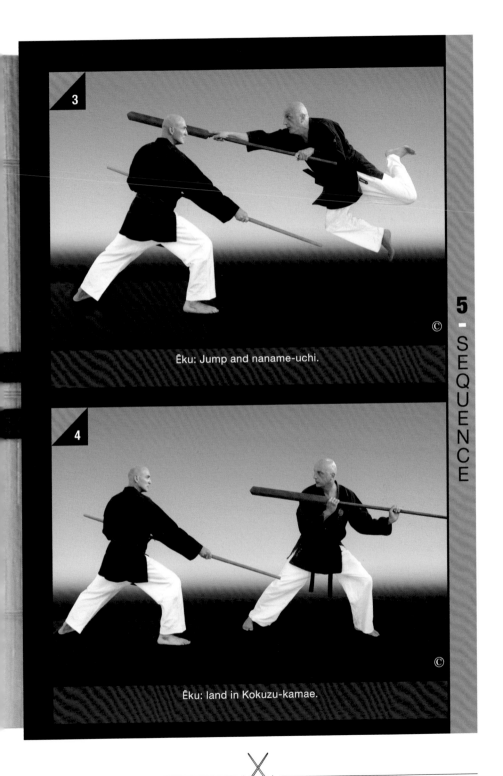

**3**

Ēku: Jump and naname-uchi.

**4**

Ēku: land in Kokuzu-kamae.

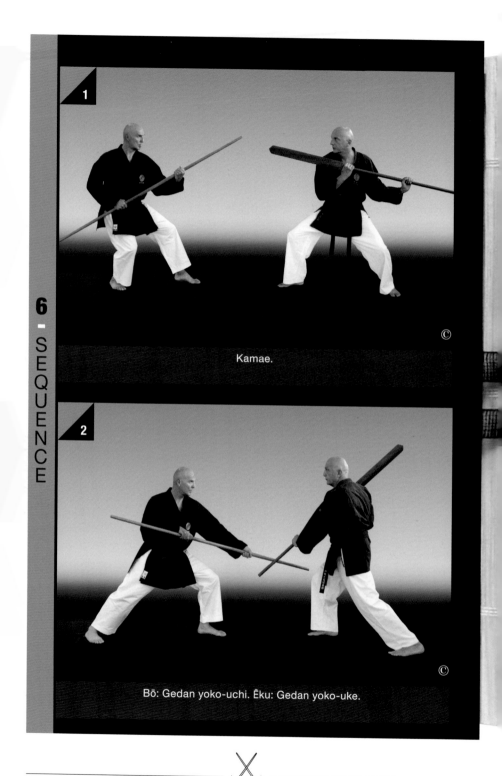

Kamae.

Bō: Gedan yoko-uchi. Êku: Gedan yoko-uke.

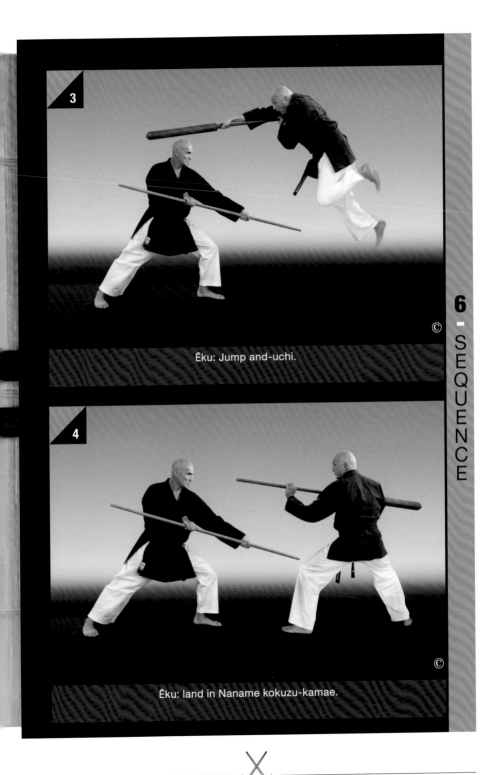

Ēku: Jump and-uchi.

Ēku: land in Naname kokuzu-kamae.

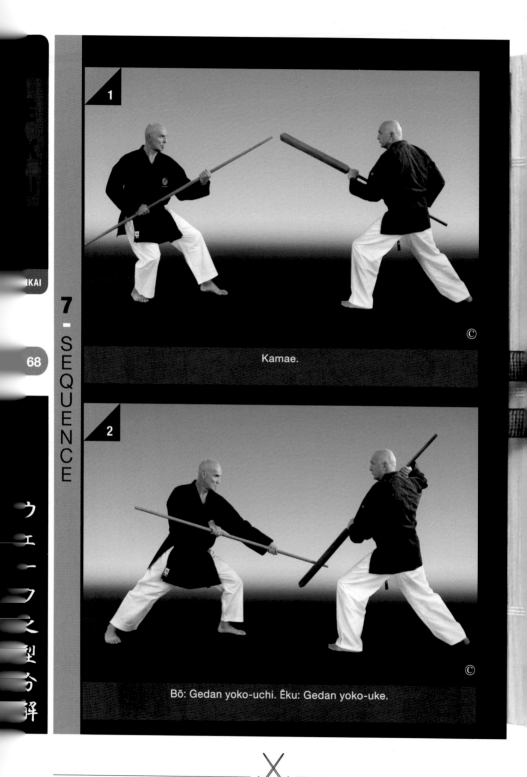

**1**

Kamae.

©

**2**

Bō: Gedan yoko-uchi. Êku: Gedan yoko-uke.

©

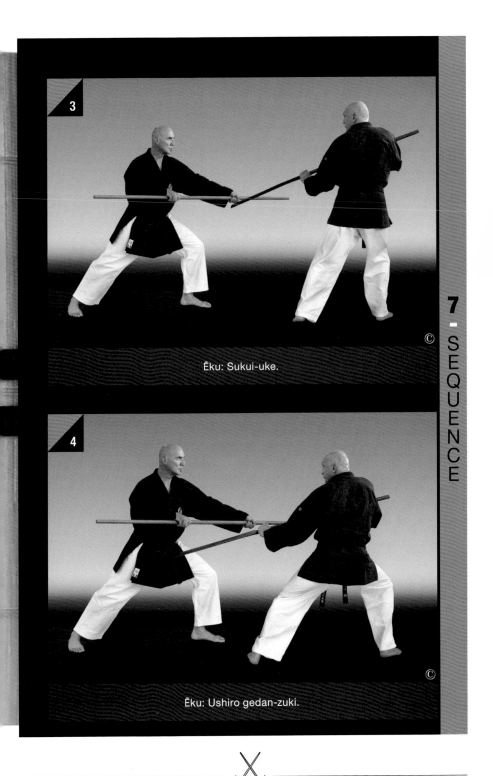

Ēku: Sukui-uke.

Ēku: Ushiro gedan-zuki.

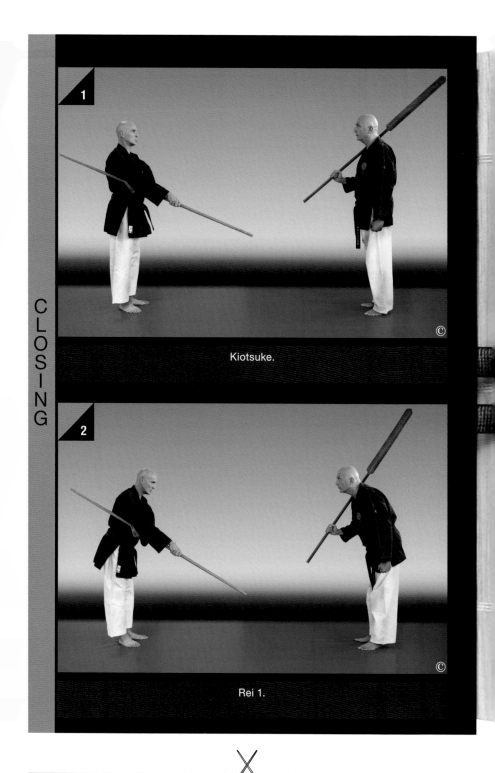

Kiotsuke.

Rei 1.

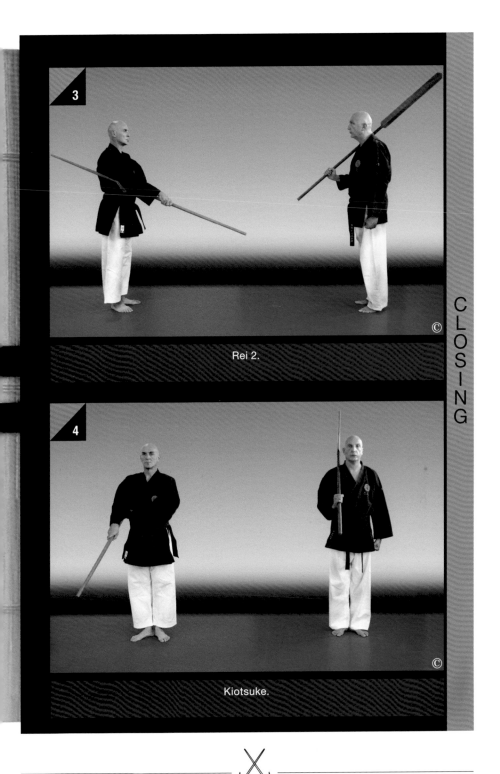

Rei 2.

Kiotsuke.

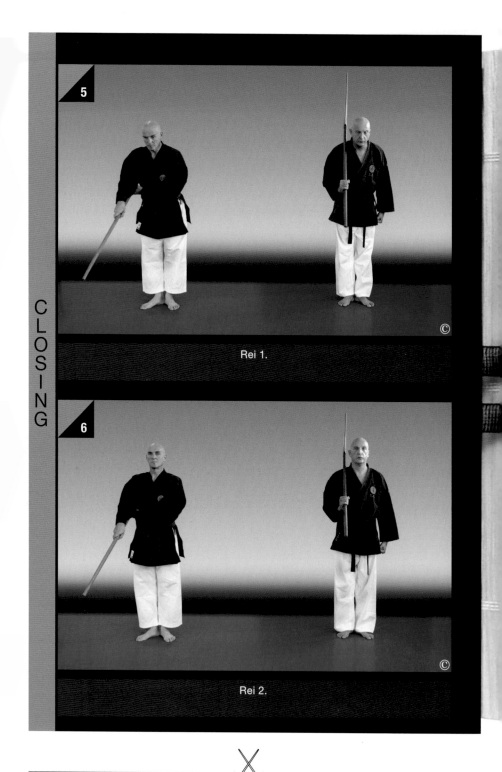

5

Rei 1.

6

Rei 2.

## FIRST SEQUENCE
**Kata techniques from 6 to 9 and 11.**

1. Kamae.
2. Bō: Jodan yoko-uchi. Ēku: Yoko-uke.
3. Ēku: Osae-uke.
4. Bō: Jodan zuki. Ēku: Gyakute kake-uke.
5. Ēku: Sunakake.
6. Ēku: Jodan kaeshi-zuki.

## SECOND SEQUENCE
**Kata techniques from 20 to 22.**

1. Kamae.
2. Bō: Gedan yoko-uchi. Ēku: Gedan yoko-uke.
3. Ēku: Naname age-uchi. Bō: Yoko-uke.
4. Ēku: Gyakute jodan-zuki.

## THIRD SEQUENCE
**Kata techniques from 36 to 41.**

1. Kamae.
2. Bō: Jodan shomen-uchi. Ēku: Jodan age-uke.
3. Ēku: Gedan yoko-uchi. Bō: raise the left leg.
4. Ēku: Ura-uchi. Bō: Yoko-uke.
5. Ēku: Kaeshi-uchi. Bō: Otoshi-uke.

6. Ēku: Jodan naname-uchi. Bō: Naname-uke.
7. Ēku: Jodan-zuki.

## FORTH SEQUENCE
**Kata techniques from 42 to 43.**

1. Kamae.
2. Ēku: prepare Sunakake.
3. Ēku: Sunakake.
4. Ēku: jump and lay in Naname kokuzu-kamae.

## FIFTH SEQUENCE
**Kata technique 44.**

1. Kamae.
2. Bō: Gedan yoko-uchi. Ēku: Gedan yoko-uke.
3. Ēku: jump and Jodan naname-uchi.
4. Ēku: lay in Kokuzu-kamae.

## SIXTH SEQUENCE
**Kata technique 45.**

1. Kamae.
2. Bō: Gedan yoko-uchi. Ēku: Gedan yoko-uke.
3. Ēku: jump and Jodan-uchi (tecnica nascosta).
4. Ēku: lay in Naname kokuzu-kamae.

## SEVENTH SEQUENCE
**Kata technique 60.**

1. Kamae.
2. Bō: Gedan yoko-uchi. Ēku: Gedan yoko-uke.
3. Ēku: Sukui-uke.
4. Ēku: Ushiro gedan-zuki.

## ABOUT THE AUTHOR

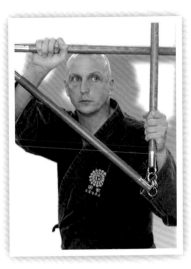

Andrea Guarelli was born in Verona, Italy, in 1961. He began practicing Karate at a young age and then added the practice of Kobudō (traditional white weapons of Okinawa, Japan).

He traveled to France frequently where many native Kobudō experts from Okinawa lived.

After several successful competitions at National level, in 1980 he was called to join the National team and he became the U.E.K. Vice European Champion and F.I.K. Team Italian Champion. In the same year the federation gave him the rank of 2° Dan and the qualification of Instructor for sport merits, he won the Panathlon award and received a merit letter to the CONI.

He qualified for the World Championship in Madrid, but he had to decline due to an injury.

In the 1980s he went to Taiwan and then to Okinawa where he trained with the Kobudō headmaster M° Shinpō Matayoshi and that of the Gōju-ryū karate Eiichi Miyazato both 10° Dan; since then he has gone to Okinawan at least once a year. In 1990 he was nominated responsible for Italy in the Zen Okinawan Kobudō Renmei (Okinawan Federation of Kobudō).

In 1993 he wrote his first articles for specialized magazines: *Quaderni d'oriente* and *Samurai*. In 1995 he organized in Bussolengo (Verona) the unique seminar in Italy of the master Shinpō Matayoshi.

In 1996 he was nominated as responsible for Italy of the Okinawan Gōju-ryū Karatedō Kyokai (Okinawan Gōju-ryū Karate Federation). In 1997 he went to Okinawa as selector for the Italian representative for the World Championship of Kobudō in Okinawa.

Master Shinpō Matayoshi gave him the rank of 6° Dan and the title of Kobudō Renshi.

In 1998 his book about the Bō of Okinawa was published by the Edizioni Mediterranee – Roma.

In 1999 he participated in Okinawa in the demonstration in honor of M° Matayoshi (anniversary of his death). In the same year he went to China (Fuzhou) where he trained with master Jin Jingfu of the White Crane.

In 2002 his book about the bō was translated in Germany by the Weinmann editor of Berlin.

In 2003 the Japanese Federation gave him the title of Karate Kyoshi. In 2008 on the occasion of a seminar in Cape Town, South African TV dedicated a service to him in the National program of martial arts "The Warrior." He went to Okinawa and China (Yongchun) where the local TV filmed him in Confucius' temple. He trained with M° Su Yinghan of the White Crane style.

The Okinawan Federation gave him the rank of 8° Dan and the title of Kobudō Kyhoshi.

In November 2009 he was nominated member of the directive council of the important association Yongchun Yiyun Society of Yongchun (Fujian – China). At the same time they gave him responsibility for the Baihequan style (White Crane) for Italy.

In 2010 he published his second book "Karatedō Nagewaza."

In 2011 during a journey to China he was invited to demonstrate a White Crane form in the temple dedicated to this style in Yong Chun, the demonstration and his interview were filmed and transmitted by TV of Taiwan. His name is engraved in the White Crane temple wall where the genealogy of this style's masters is illustrated, from the founder, Fang Qiniang, to the 12th generation which includes the author.

In September 2012 the Okinawan Federation gave him the 8° Dan of Karate.

He has taught seminars of Karate and Kobudō of Okinawa in the following countries: Spain, Germany, Denmark, Czech Republic, South Africa and USA.

He is a member of the National Association of Olympic Athletes and Italian National team members. He is the founder and president of the International Matayoshi Kobudo Association (I.M.K.A.).

Heartfelt thanks to:

My wife Fulvia.

My son Federico and my daughter Caterina.

Radana Bandovà for the creative project and the page make up of the entire volume, including photography post-production and book cover creation.

Sara Sturman for the translation.

Luca Carteri for the Japanese text translation.

Francesco Zamboni, who posed with me for the photos.

Kim Rossi Stagliano, Deux Ex Machina of the English edition.

My friend Danilo Torri.

文
武
両
道

## BIBLIOGRAPHY

- Guarelli Andrea. *Bō - Il bastone di Okinawa*, Edizioni Mediterranee - Rome - 1998
- Guarelli Andrea. *Bō - Kampf mit dem Langstock*, Weimann - Berlin - 2002
- Guarelli Andrea. *Sai-Jutsu - Il tridente di Okinawa*, Edizioni Andrea Guarelli - 2013
- Hadamitzky W. e Durmous P. *Kanji & Kana*, Edizioni J. Maisonneuve - 1984
- Hokama Tetsuhiro. *Okinawa Karate Timeline & 100 Masters*, Osato Print Co. - 2012
- Kerr George H. Okinawa. *The history of an island people*, Charles E. Tuttle Co. - 1958 e succ.
- Matayoshi Shinpō. *Ryukyu Ōchō Jidai Kobudō Karatedō*, Scritto privato - 1995
- Matayoshi Kobudō Kōdōkan. *Ko Matayoshi Shinpō Sensei Kokusai Enbu Taikai*. Kōdōkan - 1999

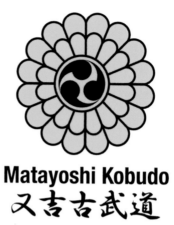

# Matayoshi Kobudo
## 又吉古武道

## TRADEMARK:

Registration n° 012649125 of 30/06/2014 by UAMI - Office of the harmonization in the internal brands, pictures and models market.

## LEGAL NOTICES:

## FURTHER INFORMATION

Anyone who is interested in the practice of the
authentic Okinawan Kobudō can contact the author
qualified teacher by consulting the A.I.K.O.
website - Associazione Italiana Kobudō di Okinawan:

**www.kobudo.it** | **book@kobudo.it**